Praise for
Hepatitis C Treatment C

"As we make prog   ....   eople in the
U.S. who have hep   ...   actical tools
and genuine hope.

—Henry C. "Hank" Johnson, Jr., U.S. Representative (D-GA),
co-chair, Congressional Viral Hepatitis Caucus

"There are many sources of information for patients to learn about hepatitis C treatment. This book is not just another of those resources. Porter's book not only provides accurate and useful information, it addresses the importance of healing mind, body, and spirit. Through her professional and personal experience with HCV, Porter is a role model for anyone ready to tackle this disease."

—Martha Saly, executive director, National Viral Hepatitis Roundtable

"Lucinda K. Porter is in a unique situation to understand the many aspects of living with hepatitis C, and this book is another generous occasion for her to share her experiences. Porter encourages patients to empower themselves with knowledge of hepatitis C and the result is a wonderful book."

—Andrew Muir, MD, Duke University

"Hepatitis C treatment is not a walk in the park but with *Hepatitis C Treatment One Step at a Time*, you have a friend to guide you down the path to living without hepatitis C."

—Lorren Sandt, executive director, Caring Ambassadors Program, Inc.

"Porter places the hepatitis C treatment into individual steps with insightful comments for daily survival, and provides the tools for individuals to reach the goal of successful treatment. With the evolution of all oral therapies for HCV by 2014 in the U.S., many parts of this book will be useful for a long time, including the advice on symptom management, advocacy, psychological, and physical preparation, and general health during treatment. Her book has brilliant insights about social preparation and financial integration with thoughtful comments on personalized medicine. Most importantly, she addresses how to overcome internal and external fears of HCV-related diseases and the treatment process. The diary structure allows readers to think about life on a day-to-day basis, and gives each patient the tools to enjoy the moment, overcome their fears, and conquer this disease."

—Robert G. Gish, MD, consultant hepatologist,
co-author of *The Hepatitis C Help Book*

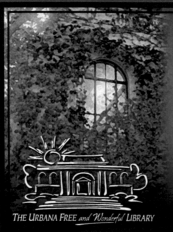

THE URBANA FREE *and Wonderful* LIBRARY

You are invited to public receptions to meet the candidates for

Library Executive Director

The Urbana Free Library Board of Trustees and the Search Committee for the Executive Director are pleased to announce that three outstanding candidates have been invited to The Urbana Free Library for on-site interviews. The public is cordially invited to meet each candidate at a scheduled reception:

Monday, February 3	Friday, February 7	Monday, February 10
Meet Celeste Choate	Meet Sarah Rosenblum	Meet Debra Stombres
4:30 to 5:30 p.m.	4:30 to 5:30 p.m.	4:30 to 5:30 p.m.
Remarks at 5:00 p.m.	Remarks at 5:00 p.m.	Remarks at 5:00 p.m.

All receptions will be held
in the MacFarlane-Hood Reading Room
on the first floor of the library.

· Light refreshments will be served ·

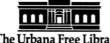

The Urbana Free Library

HEPATITIS C TREATMENT ONE STEP AT A TIME

Also by Lucinda K. Porter, RN

Free from Hepatitis C: Your Complete Guide to Healing Hepatitis C

HEPATITIS C TREATMENT ONE STEP AT A TIME

Inspiration and Practical Tips for Successful Treatment

Lucinda K. Porter, RN

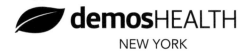

NEW YORK

Visit our website at www.demoshealth.com

ISBN: 978-1-936303-52-6
e-book ISBN: 978-1-61705-174-6

Acquisitions Editor: Julia Pastore
Compositor: diacritech

Medical information provided by Demos Health, in the absence of a visit with a health care professional, must be considered as an educational service only. This book is not designed to replace a physician's independent judgment about the appropriateness or risks of a procedure or therapy for a given patient. Our purpose is to provide you with information that will help you make your own health care decisions.

The information and opinions provided here are believed to be accurate and sound, based on the best judgment available to the authors, editors, and publisher, but readers who fail to consult appropriate health authorities assume the risk of injuries. The publisher is not responsible for errors or omissions. The editors and publisher welcome any reader to report to the publisher any discrepancies or inaccuracies noticed.

Library of Congress Cataloging-in-Publication Data

Porter, Lucinda K.

Hepatitis C treatment one step at a time: inspiration and practical tips for successful treatment / Lucinda K. Porter, RN.
     pages cm
Includes bibliographical references and index.
ISBN 978-1-936303-52-6
1. Hepatitis C—Treatment. 2. Hepatitis C—Patients—Prayers and devotions. I. Title.
RC848.H425P66 2013
616.3'62306—dc23

                                        2013028037

Special discounts on bulk quantities of Demos Health books are available to corporations, professional associations, pharmaceutical companies, health care organizations, and other qualifying groups. For details, please contact:

Special Sales Department
Demos Medical Publishing, LLC
11 West 42nd Street, 15th Floor
New York, NY 10036
Phone: 800-532-8663 or 212-683-0072
Fax: 212-941-7842
E-mail: specialsales@demosmedpub.com

Printed in the United States of America by Edwards Brothers.

13 14 15 16 17 / 5 4 3 2 1

To my father, D.E.W. Kressly, who reached lofty heights, one step at a time.

CONTENTS

Foreword by Diana L. Sylvestre, MD   xi
Author's Note   xiii
Preface   xv
Introduction   xvii

1 How to Use This Book   *1*

2 Preparing for Treatment   *5*

3 Readings for the First 12 Weeks   *17*

4 Readings for Weeks 13 through 24   *65*

5 Readings for Weeks 25 through 36   *111*

6 Readings for the Final 12 Weeks   *155*

7 Waiting for Results   *195*

8 When Treatment Doesn't Work   *199*

Conclusion   *203*
Appendix A: Foods with 20 Grams of Fat   *205*
Appendix B: Managing Anal/Rectal Discomfort   *207*
Appendix C: Managing Skin Problems   *209*
Resources   *211*
Acknowledgments   *219*
Index   *221*

FOREWORD

These days, it's hard to do anything in the field of hepatitis C without hearing about Lucinda Porter. As if her prior book *Free from Hepatitis C: Your Complete Guide to Healing Hepatitis C* weren't enough, she maintains several blogs and two monthly columns in the *HCV Advocate*. There are speaking engagements and lectures and even a TEDx talk. What is it with her, has she cloned herself?

Don't get me wrong, I think this is terrific. I run the OASIS Clinic in Oakland, California, a little clinic recognized for showing that people who are supposedly "untreatable" can successfully complete treatment just like everyone else. The key is to provide the right kind of education and support. Our mantra is: If one of us has hepatitis C, all of us have it. It doesn't matter who you are or how you got it, the more you know about hepatitis C the better your outcomes will be.

That is why having Lucinda in our community is a Really Good Thing. Both of us being strong proponents of self-advocacy and education, I've known her for years. But Lucinda isn't just a nurse and outstanding educator; she herself has hepatitis C and has also gone through the challenging treatment three times. She writes as both a treater and a patient, and knows how important support is to being successful in hepatitis C.

This is a gem of a book, filled with bite-sized pieces of information to step you through the treatment process. It is like a friendly little companion. There are daily motivational readings and tips; the journey begins before you start treatment, stays with you each day you are taking medications, and helps you after it is over as well. It remains hopeful about success but will help you manage if the treatment doesn't work. The messages are accessible and brief and thoughtful. The main problem is this: you are going to want to cheat and read ahead!

The landscape of hepatitis C treatment is changing, and treatment will get easier and more effective in the coming years. But we are not there yet and not everyone can wait. If you need treatment for your hepatitis C, it will be a challenge but you can do it. You must prepare yourself and get the education and support you need. I think you will find this lovely book will help you reach that goal.

Diana L. Sylvestre, MD
Executive Director, OASIS Clinic
Co-Author, *Healing Hepatitis C*
Oakland, California

AUTHOR'S NOTE

Your medical provider may be a physician, nurse, or physician's assistant. Throughout this book, I use the term *medical provider* when referring to these professionals.

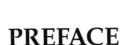

PREFACE

Those who would climb to a lofty height must go by steps, not leaps.
—St. Gregory the Great

When I wrote the main body of this book, I did not know that I would be starting my own treatment for hepatitis C. As I write these words, I am experiencing some of what my readers will be facing—side effects, questions, and an unsettled world. This is my third time through hepatitis C treatment, so I may not be feeling as anxious as you are, particularly if you are embarking on treatment for the first (and I hope the last) time.

As both a hepatitis C nurse and patient, I have accumulated a mountain of information and tips for successful management of hepatitis C treatment. My first book, *Free from Hepatitis C,* is a guide to help patients through hepatitis C, from diagnosis through treatment. The book that you are holding in your hands, *Hepatitis C Treatment One Step at a Time,* is a toolkit packed with daily tips and encouraging words to help you reach the goal of successful treatment. I would describe my first book as a "how-to" manual. This book is more like a coach, telling you how to cope with treatment while suggesting strategies for your success.

So here we are, each beginning our journey, separate yet together. May your road be easy and your side effects light. Most of all, may you reach the finish line safely. The only way to do this is one step at a time. I'll see you at the finish line!

INTRODUCTION

Whatever you can do or dream you can, begin it. Boldness has genius, power, and magic in it!

—*Johann Wolfgang von Goethe*

Hepatitis C virus (HCV) is the most common blood-borne infection in the United States. The Centers for Disease Control and Prevention (CDC) states that 3.2 million Americans are infected with HCV; some experts point out that because the CDC didn't survey people with high risk for HCV, estimates are closer to five million or more. Of those who have it, 75 percent are baby boomers born from 1946 through 1965. Since 2007, more people in the United States have died from HCV than from HIV. The majority of those who have HCV are unaware that they have it.

Unless something is done, the death rate from HCV is expected to rise. HCV damages the liver slowly, often taking more than 20 years before its impact is noticeable. At its worst, HCV can cause severe scarring of the liver, a condition known as *cirrhosis*. Those with cirrhosis are at risk for liver cancer, end-stage liver disease, and death. The symptoms of cirrhosis include accumulation of fluid in the belly (*ascites*), risk of hemorrhage, and a heartbreaking dementia known as *hepatic encephalopathy*. Experts estimate that by 2020, more than a million people with HCV will have cirrhosis in the United States.

Even those without cirrhosis may be suffering from the effects of this virus. HCV multiplies a trillion times a day in the liver, causing liver damage and various symptoms. Fatigue is the most common complaint, but depression, and cognitive problems are frequently reported. Because the body's immune system tries to destroy HCV, patients may experience muscle and joint pains, headaches, and dry mouth. Sometimes other organs are affected and people with HCV are at higher risk for other diseases and death from causes other than just from liver-related ones.

For many, the emotional burden that accompanies HCV can be worse than the physical one. HCV has the power to rob hope from the future. Patients wonder what this virus will do to them, their families, and their dreams. Fear of infecting others is a frequent burden, as patients obsess over whether they have done all they can to protect those with whom they come in contact. Finally, there is HCV's stigma, brought on both because of having an infectious virus, and its association with injection drug use. For some, HCV's stigma is a heavier burden than the virus is.

As one of the millions with HCV, I understand what it is like to live with it. I acquired HCV during a blood transfusion in 1988, when the virus was still known as *non-A, non-B hepatitis*. The blood transfusion saved my life; hepatitis C changed my life. Fear about having HCV, suffering with it, and perhaps dying from it crippled me more than the virus did. In time, I learned to live without fear. The great paradox is that HCV has given me a new enthusiasm for life. Living with a life-threatening virus is a dramatic reminder to get the most out of today, since nobody knows what tomorrow will bring. Now, hepatitis C is not merely a diagnosis to me; it is my calling.

HCV treatment has a reputation for being a grueling therapy, which at times it is. Some people have easy experiences; some are really tested. Since 1997, I have worked with HCV patients in various communities across North America. At Stanford University Medical Center, I was on a team with some of the top physicians in the field of liver disease, and although I credit them with teaching me a great deal, it was the patients who taught me the most. Many patients discovered that treatment wasn't as bad as they thought it would be, and being extraordinary is not a requirement to make it to the finish line.

I have been through HCV treatment twice, and am now going through it again. The first treatment was in 1997, when the only option was interferon alfa, a protein given by self-injection to stimulate the immune system. Interferon occurs in the body naturally, produced when needed to fight a cold, virus, or other microorganism. The achy feeling you get when you are coming down with something is actually from interferon rather than from the invading virus.

Because I have a hard-to-treat variation of the virus (genotype 1a), my chances of responding were low. I stopped after three months, since interferon alone was not enough to give HCV the boot. In late 2002, I underwent a 48-week course of treatment using two drugs—peginterferon and ribavirin. Peginterferon (Pegasys or PegIntron) is a more durable form of interferon. Ribavirin (Rebetol, Copegus, and Ribasphere) is a pill that weakens HCV. This treatment combination gave me a 50 percent chance of permanently eliminating HCV.

Unfortunately, although I cleared HCV, once I completed the medications, the virus came back. Even though I wasn't cured, I benefited from treatment. Like most who do treatment, my liver had the opportunity to do some quality repair work as it got a break from

Genotypes

Genotypes are genetic variations of HCV.

There are six genotypes:1, 2, 3, 4, 5, 6.

Most HCV genotypes have subtypes. For instance, those with genotype 1 have either 1a or 1b.

Some genotypes respond to treatment more easily, particularly genotypes 2 and 3. Genotype 1 is the most common genotype in the Unites States. It is the hardest to treat, so usually three drugs are used for those with genotype 1, whereas genotype 2 and 3 patients only take two drugs. The subtype 1b responds to current medications more easily than 1a.

HCV's constant assault. My liver biopsy showed significant improvement as a result.

Treatment success rates are now around 80 percent. Patients with genotype 2, 3, and even some genotype 1 patients have shorter treatment durations of 24 or 28 weeks. Although others may need up to 48 weeks of treatment, this is usually determined after 12 weeks. Information gathered at this stage may also determine that it is best to stop altogether.

Patients with genotype 2 or 3 still take the medications that have been in use since 2002—peginterferon and ribavirin. Genotype 1 patients are treated with those two drugs, plus an additional pill called a *protease inhibitor*, either boceprevir (Victrelis) or telaprevir (Incivek). A small percentage of patients have other genotypes, and they usually are treated with peginterferon and ribavirin for varying durations.

Many new drugs are in the pipeline, and at least two are expected to be approved by 2014. The U.S. Food and Drug Administration (FDA) granted priority review to Janssen's simeprevir and Gilead's sofosbuvir. If approved, simeprevir is for genotype 1 patients. It is a daily pill taken with peginterferon and ribavirin.

If sofosbuvir is approved, patients with genotype 1, 4, 5 and 6 who have had no prior HCV treatment, may have the option to take sofosbuvir in combination with peginterferon and ribavirin. Genotype 2 and 3 patients may have a chance at an all-oral HCV treatment, combining sofosbuvir with ribavirin. However, the treatment response rates for genotype 3 patients were significantly lower than genotype 2, so this group may have better odds with peginterferon and ribavirin.

Now I am back at my third treatment. HCV has compromised my ability to get health insurance, so I have elected to participate in a clinical trial. With current treatment rates at 80 percent and above, I realize that I am risking the better odds that come with triple-therapy, but it is the option I can afford. If the test drugs don't work, then when I get insurance under the Patient Protection and Affordable Care Act, I can try something else.

It may sound like I am a strong person, but I am not. If tortured, I'd spill national security secrets if my captors threatened to cut my fingernails short, let alone pull them out. After reading about HCV medication side effects, I seriously doubted my ability to make it through, particularly since I am practically phobic about vomiting. However, I was surprised—HCV treatment was not as bad as I had imagined it would be, and I got through it.

Perhaps I am not a poster child for HCV treatment, since I have not been cured yet. However, I am a poster child for believing that we can be cured. You, me, we can beat HCV. One of the myths about HCV is that it is not treatable or curable. The majority of HCV patients can be treated, and the medications keep getting better. HCV treatment rates are at their highest. Medical providers are tailoring patients' treatment plans by using *response-guided therapy*. Patients who meet certain requirements, including an early and rapid response to the HCV medications, may qualify for shorter lengths of treatment, and less treatment means fewer side effects. If HCV is successfully eliminated for more than six months after completing antiviral therapy, the odds that it will return are about one half of one percent.

The odds are in our favor. If you join me in this journey, it will help to have the tools that I have. This book provides tips and motivation to stay on course. If you are ready to start, here is your first tip: add a healthy dose of hope to your toolbox. Christopher Reeve said, "Once you choose hope, anything's possible." Yes, anything is possible, including curing hepatitis C.

1

How to Use this Book

Once you make a decision, the universe conspires to make it happen.
                                            —Ralph Waldo Emerson

This book provides daily readings to help you stay motivated and tips to help you through HCV treatment. It is meant to be a companion who whispers in your ear, "you can do this," while providing guidelines to help you reach your goal.

Despite the fact that there are millions of people with HCV, no two patients are alike and treatment is tailored to accommodate these differences. With response-guided therapy, the length of your treatment will likely be 24, 28, 36, or 48 weeks. A small subset of patients may have shorter or longer treatment duration. This book is designed to meet these variations.

Start with the chapter "Preparing for Treatment." This chapter provides words of comfort, and inspiration to address common issues that may arise as you prepare for treatment. When it is time to start taking the medication, begin with "Readings for the First 12 Weeks." The day of your first injection will line up with week 1, day 1 in this chapter. If your treatment is exactly 48 weeks, then just follow this book as it is written.

If you started treatment before reading this book, pick up at the point where you are in your treatment. I recommend reading the material you missed, particularly the earliest entries, as they provide a foundation for successful treatment. The readings are short, and you may acquire information to ease your treatment experience.

If your treatment plan is shorter than 48 weeks, modify the readings to fit your regimen. For instance, if your treatment is twelve weeks, read the first 12 weeks as well as the last week. Since the readings are short, you could read both the first and last twelve weeks simultaneously. If your medical provider prescribes 28 weeks of treatment, read "Readings for the First 12 Weeks," 4 weeks from "Readings for Weeks 13 through 24," and finish with "Readings for the Final 12 Weeks."

HCV treatment rarely exceeds 48 weeks, but should this happen, you can double up on your readings or use the index to locate information about a particular issue. Focus on ending your treatment with the readings provided for the final 12 weeks and the variations will handle themselves.

Some of the readings and tips may seem redundant. There is a reason for this. Some things can't be said often enough. However, each reading offers something new to help you gain mastery over HCV treatment.

When you complete treatment, go to the "Waiting for Results" chapter. The odds are in your favor that treatment will work, but if it does not, you will wonder what to do next. If that happens, or if your medical provider stops treatment early because the medications aren't working, go to the chapter entitled "When Treatment Doesn't Work."

If at any point you are discontinuing treatment because the medications are not working or side effects force you to quit, skip to Chapter 8, "When Treatment Doesn't Work." If you discontinue early but don't know the results yet, you can read Chapter 7, "Waiting for Results."

Although the index will help you find information pertaining to specific issues that may arise, three appendices provide important information. Appendix A is a list of foods containing 20 grams of fat, which those taking telaprevir will need to eat when taking their pills. The other appendices include information on two side effects, anal/ rectal discomfort and skin problems. These two common side effects can cause a lot of misery, which can be avoided with early, proactive management.

For those wanting more information, the Resources guide provides links to various organizations. The Internet is a huge, sometimes overwhelming place, and these listed resources are reliable. Resources can also help you locate a support group or assistance with patient advocacy. Perhaps you want current information about HCV. If so, look under "Hepatitis C and HIV/HCV Co-Infection Information." The "Blogs and News" section will lead you to people writing about HCV, including me.

Part of successful HCV treatment includes access to health insurance and dealing with disability if it becomes difficult to work during this time. Two sections will help with these: "Disability, Disclosure, and Workplace Issues" and "Financial Issues and Medical Insurance." If you do not have medical insurance, then you may be interested in the "Clinical Trial" section.

I strongly urge looking under the "Pharmaceutical Companies" heading to take advantage of the tools and support provided by the manufacturer of the HCV treatment drugs you are taking. Take advantage of the savings plans that the pharmaceutical companies offer.

As you receive information about your treatment progress, you may want to learn more about lab tests, so a section is provided. Although this book focuses primarily on HCV treatment side effects, new information is always coming into view, so you may want to look at the links provided under "Side Effects." Be sure to visit the Hep Drug Interactions website listed in this section.

Throughout the book, I promote basic health practices. You will find links to these under the following headings: "Brain Fitness," "Nutrition," "Physical Fitness," and "Sleep." There is good information under the broader subject, "General Health and Health Improvement." For those interested in complementary and alternative medicine, there is a section for you.

If you or a loved one struggles with alcohol or drugs, there are links to help under the category, "Substance Abuse and Recovery." Mental health links are listed in a section. For those taking antidepressant medication using selective serotonin reuptake inhibitors (SSRIs), there is excellent information about these medications on the Mayo Clinic site. If you are looking for help with anger management, stress relief, or wanting more peace in your life, look under "Meditation, Stress Reduction, and Anger Management."

If it has been awhile since you have practiced birth control, look under "Pregnancy and Contraception." You can also find information about "Hepatitis C Transmission and Prevention."

The two categories that I hope everyone uses are "Humor" and "Storytelling." Humor will lift your spirits and keep you on track. Storytelling is what we do to connect with others. We find hope by hearing others' stories; we heal when we tell our own. We all have stories to tell, and now yours is about to begin a new chapter.

2

Preparing for Treatment

It is better to look ahead and prepare than to look back and regret.
—Jackie Joyner-Kersee

Treatment is like a marathon race—advanced preparation is critical to successful completion. This chapter suggests ways you can prepare yourself physically, mentally, and emotionally for this big event.

LEARN EVERYTHING YOU CAN ABOUT HCV TREATMENT

Success depends upon previous preparation, and without such preparation, there is sure to be failure.
—Confucius

Discuss HCV Treatment Options with Your Medical Provider. In addition to resources, your provider is the one who should have answers to your questions.

- What are the pros and cons of treatment?
- What medications does your medical provider suggest for you?
- How are the medications taken? If one of the medications is injectable, will you need to give it to yourself? If so, will you be shown how to do this?

- Are there any special storage requirements for the HCV drugs?
- What are the most common side effects?
- How long will treatment last?
- How is it determined that treatment is or is not working, and when will you know?
- How often are the lab tests and medical appointments?
- Will you need a liver biopsy or other diagnostic tests?
- Will treatment affect your work? Your relationships? Your sex life?
- How much will treatment cost? Are there financial assistance programs available to help reduce out-of-pocket costs?
- Are there any drugs, herbs, or supplements that may interact with the HCV treatment medications?
- What immunizations does your medical provider recommend, and are you up-to-date on these?
- Are there any hepatitis C groups in the area?
- What do you do if you miss a dose of medication?
- If you need support from your medical provider during treatment, who do you contact in the office, especially after regular business hours?
- Is there a list of side effects that may require urgent medical attention? If not, what are some situations in which you should call your provider immediately? Here is a list of medical problems that may need emergency care:
  - Chest pain
  - Breathing difficulties
  - Dizziness
  - Severe depression, thoughts of harming yourself or others, and mania (periods of very high moods followed by very low moods)
  - A persistent fever over 100°F or fever that continues to elevate
  - Vision changes—double, blurred, and decreased or loss of vision
  - Bloody diarrhea
  - Unusual bleeding or bruising
  - Severe pain in your stomach or lower back
  - Weakness, loss of coordination, numbness, or difficulty speaking
  - A rash with fever, blisters, swelling, or sores in the mouth, nose, or eyes
  - Hearing loss
  - Any symptom that might be potentially life threatening or causes excessive anxiety

Speak to Others Who Have Undergone Treatment. You can find people to talk to at hepatitis C groups in your area. If there are no groups, consider a web-based group. You can also ask your medical provider if he or she can pass your name along to other patients if they want to contact you. Your medical provider cannot disclose other patients' names, but you can give permission to disclose yours. Also, you might be surprised at how many people in your community have experience with HCV treatment. I live in a small town, and I know many people who are treatment-experienced or have a family member or friend who is. If you talk about having HCV, others will often open up about it.

Read as Much as You Can About Treatment. There are some excellent websites and publications about hepatitis C. Here is a list of my top recommendations:

- HCV Advocate (www.hcvadvocate.org): There are hundreds of free factsheets and guides to help you with HCV. Topics cover a huge range, including stigma, lab tests, workplace issues, and so forth. If you want basic information, read *Understanding HCV: A Patient's Pocket Guide* or look in the section "The Basics of HCV." Guides that may be particularly beneficial during treatment are: *A Guide to Hepatitis C: Preparing for Treatment*; *A Guide to Hepatitis C: Treatment Side Effect Management*; and *HCV Treatment: A Guide to Help You Stay on Treatment*. For those who are co-infected with HIV, I suggest *HIV and Hepatitis Co-infections: Management and Treatment Guidelines*.
- *Free from Hepatitis C: Your Complete Guide to Healing Hepatitis C* I wrote this to help patients navigate HCV treatment and side effect management.
- For information on HCV treatment and related subjects, browse the recommended links in the Resources guide at the back of this book.

CONFRONT FEAR

I have learned over the years that when one's mind is made up, this diminishes fear; knowing what must be done does away with fear.
—Rosa Parks

Pretty much everyone is afraid before they start HCV treatment. You may be wondering all sorts of things, such as what side effects will you get and if you can handle them. How will the drugs make you feel? Will they work? Will you be able to work? What will this do to your relationships? Will you be a good mother, father, partner, employee, boss, caregiver, and so on, during this time?

Hundreds of thousands of people have gone through treatment, and I bet most were afraid. I wish I could say something that would make the fear go away, but I can't. What I can tell you is that for me and everyone I talked to, fear diminishes after you start treatment. It's like standing on a diving board for the first time, wondering if you are going to break your neck on the pool bottom. Encouraging words don't remove the dread; it is the act of jumping in that reveals how unnecessary the anxiety was in the first place. Acknowledge the fear, and then try to focus on doing everything you can for a successful treatment experience.

PREPARE YOUR BODY

I teach you to preserve your health so that you will succeed better in proportion as you avoid doctors.
—*Leonardo da Vinci*

Your body will be the vessel that bears the majority of side effects. Aim for getting your body in top form before you begin and then do your best to maintain this level of health. If you don't have much time before starting treatment, you can implement changes in the early stages. Here are some important considerations to maximize your health and treatment experience:

- Rule out pregnancy for you or your partner prior to starting HCV medications, and have a birth control plan. During treatment and for six months after completion, use two forms of contraception between you and your partner, unless pregnancy is not possible. (These medications may cause fetal abnormalities or death, so be sure to read the warning that accompanies these drugs.) If you have questions about birth control or the Ribavirin Pregnancy Registry, see the "Pregnancy and Conception" section in Resources at the back of this book.
- Make sure you have all pretreatment lab tests, including viral load and genotype tests.
- Be sure you are up-to-date on your immunizations, including hepatitis A and B, flu, and tetanus. Your medical provider may also recommend shingles and pneumonia vaccinations. It is okay to get these during treatment if that is the earliest you can do at this time.
- Since HCV medications may cause eye-related side effects, have a baseline ophthalmic exam before you start treatment.
- If you are planning to have any elective medical or dental procedures, try to schedule these prior to or early in treatment.

- Because HCV treatment may lower the "feel good" hormones in the brain, some medical providers recommend using antidepressant medication during HCV treatment. See if your provider wants you to start antidepressants before you take the HCV drugs or to wait and see if you need them. If you are already taking antidepressants, your medical provider may suggest modifying your current medications.
- Avoid alcohol and other chemical substances before, during, and after HCV treatment.
- Make regular physical activity a habit. Walking, swimming, bicycling, dancing, weight training, stretching, yoga, tai chi, Pilates, gardening, and playing with children or a dog are some good choices since you can do these throughout treatment. Regular physical activity can be done in short intervals throughout the day.

PREPARE YOUR MIND

A strong positive mental attitude will create more miracles than any wonder drug.
—Patricia Neal

Although your body will bear the brunt of treatment, it is crucial that you prepare your mind for what is to come. Try to cultivate a positive attitude because a negative one can worsen your treatment experience. HCV medications will affect your moods. Striving to remain positive may give you an edge, by helping to combat those sour moods that aren't medication-induced.

Before you begin, remind yourself that difficulties and delays may lie ahead. If you could see them clearly, naturally, you would do a great deal to get rid of them, but you can't. You can only see one thing clearly, and that is your goal of becoming free of HCV. Form a mental image of that goal and cling to it.

Saturate your environment with reminders to help you stay on course. Post encouraging words on your computer screensaver, cell phone, and mirror. This book provides quotes for every day. If you find a quote that shores you up, make a note of it. Here are some to get you started:

Acceptance of the unacceptable is the greatest source of grace in this world.
—Eckhart Tolle

But screw your courage to the sticking-place and we'll not fail.
—William Shakespeare

Courage is being scared to death but saddling up anyway.
—John Wayne

Courage is the discovery that you may not win, and trying when you know you can lose.

—Tom Krause

Courage is the price that life exacts for granting peace. The soul that knows it not, knows no release from little things; knows not the livid loneliness of fear.

—Amelia Earhart

If there is no struggle, there is no progress.

—Frederick Douglass

If you can't change your fate, change your attitude.

—Amy Tan

I must be willing to give up what I am in order to become what I will be.

—Albert Einstein

Life loves to be taken by the lapel and told: I'm with you kid. Let's go.
—Maya Angelou

Of one thing I am certain, the body is not the measure of healing—peace is the measure.

—George Melton

The more serious the illness, the more important it is for you to fight back, mobilizing all your resources—spiritual, emotional, intellectual, physical. Your heaviest artillery will be your will to live. Keep that big gun going.

—Norman Cousins

This is no time for ease and comfort. It is the time to dare and endure.
—Winston Churchill

CULTIVATE HUMOR

A person without a sense of humor is like a wagon without springs—jolted by every pebble on the road.

—Henry Ward Beecher

Laughter can make just about anything better, unless you just had stomach surgery or your jaw wired. Find ways to laugh on a daily basis. Start collecting jokes, comic strips, inspiring or humorous literature, videos, and websites. Subscribe to daily jokes on the Internet or buy a joke-a-day calendar. Surround yourself with friends who make you laugh. Check out my blog, *The Hepatitis Comics: Levity for the Liver* at hepatitiscomics.blogspot.com. If you make humor a priority, you will find it all around you.

BE GRATEFUL

So much has been given to me; I have no time to ponder over that which has been denied.

—Helen Keller

Gratitude is an effective tool against a poor attitude. Every day, make a list of at least three things for which you are grateful. Here are three examples:

- I am grateful for the latest advances in HCV treatment.
- I am grateful that I have medical care.
- I am grateful for this chance to get rid of HCV.

FEED YOUR SPIRIT

When you examine the lives of the most influential people who have ever walked among us, you discover one thread that winds through them all. They have been aligned first with their spiritual nature and only then with their physical selves.

—Albert Einstein

The realm of the spirit is deeply personal. If you are pulled by spiritual matters, there is no time like the present to strengthen your spiritual practice.

Meditation and prayer are the mainstays of spiritual practice. Research shows that meditation lowers blood pressure, reduces pain, and improves certain skin conditions, such as psoriasis. Meditation also helps with anxiety, depression, and sleep problems. Increased immune function and improved sex lives are some other benefits of this simple practice. Hildegard of Bingen described prayer as "breathing in and breathing out the one breath of the Universe." Whether you call it prayer or meditation, devote time every day to being aware of your breath, and you may be surprised at the results.

GET ORGANIZED

Order is the sanity of the mind, the health of the body, the peace of the city, the security of the state. Like beams in a house or bones to a body, so is order to all things.

—Robert Southey

There is quite a lot to keep track of—everything from taking pills on time to juggling medical appointments. Taking your pills on time is hugely important, particularly if you are taking boceprevir, telaprevir, or similar drug(s) classified as HCV Direct Antiviral Agents (DAAs). DAAs are like antibiotics in that each time you miss a dose, there is a risk that the virus will build resistance, making it more difficult to treat.

A reminder system will help you manage your treatment, and here are tools to help you:

- Use pill organizers. If you have to take pills three times a day, get three organizers or one that has three compartments per day.
- Devise a system for remembering to take your medication, and stick to it.
- Use a calendar to write down all your appointments and reminders to get labs and refill prescriptions.
- Keep a notepad and write everything down, even if you think you will remember it. Jotting down your errands, shopping list, and phone calls to make maximizes your chances of maintaining the structure of your life without the additional frustration that accompanies forgetfulness.
- Use electronic devices, such as phone, computer, e-mail, or voicemail to remind you to take your medications, attend appointments, and refill prescriptions. If you have a smart phone, reminder apps such as *GenieMD* are a huge help.
- Store things such as keys, wallet, purse, checkbook, cellular phone, and other items in the same place each day and you won't need to look for them.
- Organize your health records. Ask for copies of lab results and other tests, such as liver biopsy reports. Keep everything in one place, such as a notebook, file cabinet, computer, or a box. If you store information on your computer or mobile device, make sure you back it up.

PREPARE OTHERS

We are all dependent on one another, every soul of us on earth.
                                                              —George Bernard Shaw

HCV treatment doesn't just affect you; it affects others. Even if you are able to maintain your daily activities, it will be apparent that you are not feeling well. You may be tired, short-tempered, or distracted. If you live or interact with others on a regular basis, it is best to tell them the cause of this change in you. If you don't want to tell them the exact details, you can simply say that you are undergoing a treatment for a blood disorder, a treatment that has many side effects including ones that might affect your usual demeanor. You can reassure them that this is temporary and not life threatening.

A benefit of being open about your treatment is that it invites clear communication. Those who are close to you may feel helpless about your disease and its treatment. The ability to talk about it may reduce their feelings of helplessness. You can involve others in your treatment by giving them literature to read, inviting them to appointments, and soliciting their help by reminding you to take your medication, if this is useful to you.

Some people are more private and prefer that others keep out of their medical affairs. If this is your style, then ask those around you to respect this. Consider meeting them halfway by keeping them informed of your progress, and reassuring them that you will tell them if they need to be concerned about your health. Let them know that you appreciate their interest.

Workplace disclosure is a bit trickier. Despite our best efforts, side effects are difficult to hide. If your work or mood is affected, this may be noticed by co-workers or your supervisor. In certain employment situations, you are protected under the Americans with Disabilities Act (ADA). To receive this protection, you must disclose that you have a medical problem. Your employer is supposed to protect your privacy, but the reality is that people talk. You may want to keep the details of your illness and treatment vague, supplying just enough to allow protection under the ADA.

SET UP A SUPPORT SYSTEM

No one is rich enough to do without a neighbor.
—*Danish Proverb*

If you do nothing else to prepare for this treatment, find an HCV group. The term *support group* may conjure up images of people sitting around dabbing their eyes with tissue, a myth that needs correction. HCV groups are usually information-based, and a good group is usually filled with laughter, not tears. There are community and Internet-based groups. Find one that meets your needs. There are many fine hepatitis C organizations that offer support in various ways, but a good one to turn to is *Help4Hep*. Its website and phone number are listed in Resources.

The support of family and friends is also important, as well as that of your community. Perhaps you already have a strong support system in place for purposes other than HCV. If you attend a church, a recovery program, clubs, or other organizations that bring value, strength, or just plain fun to your life, continue to attend these. If you feel comfortable revealing the fact that you are undergoing HCV treatment to those who are closest to you, this may provide another avenue of support.

Other sources of support include your medical team, pharmacy, and the pharmaceutical companies who manufacture HCV medications. Some pharmaceutical companies offer 24-hour phone service, literature, and web-based support. These usually offer high-quality information and can be extremely valuable.

FINANCIAL PREPARATIONS

A nickel isn't worth a dime today.

—Yogi Berra

HCV treatment is very costly. Before you begin, make sure your insurance covers the medications. Find out what your co-pay and deductible are. If the drugs are not covered, see if you qualify for financial assistance or a clinical trial.

Some people may need to take time off from work during treatment. If or when this happens is primarily determined by how you react to the medications and the type of work you do. For instance, if you are a roofer and the medications make you dizzy, then you may need to take sick leave. Some people may have the option to modify their work, so a roofer who can answer phones in an office might still be able to work. Look into your employer's sick leave and disability provisions. If you are self-employed or do not have medical coverage, be sure you can afford time off should it become necessary.

KNOW YOUR PROTOCOL

The person who is well prepared has already won half of the battle.

—Portuguese Proverb

Hepatitis C treatment is complicated. There are various medications, and the regimens for each are guided by a variety of factors, such as genotype, previous treatment response, the presence of cirrhosis, and the patient's response to the current regimen. Additionally, medical providers may each have their own way of administering these protocols.

Before you begin, ask your medical provider to map out your protocol. You may not know the length of your treatment, but you certainly should know the worst- and best-case scenarios and have a timeline for lab tests. Spend some time reading about lab testing, either by looking over your medication's package insert or online resources for "HCV Treatment Algorithm." If your medical provider suggests a protocol that differs from what you read, ask for an explanation.

Be sure you are not taking drugs, dietary supplements, and over-the-counter medications that may interact with HCV medications. Tell your medical provider everything you are taking, particularly if your treatment includes a direct-acting antiviral, such as boceprevir or telaprevir. For instance, the dosage for erectile dysfunction drugs (tadalafil/Cialis, sildenafil/Viagra, and vardenafil/Levitra) may need to be reduced when taking boceprevir or telaprevir. The dose for the sleep agent, zolpidem (Ambien), may need to be increased. You should not take the herb St. John's wort while taking boceprevir or telaprevir. The list of drug interactions can be found online or in the package insert that accompanies your medication. You can also check for potential interactions by using the Hep Drug Interactions website listed under *Side Effects*.

PREPARE FOR SIDE EFFECTS

If you want the rainbow, you gotta put up with the rain.
—Dolly Parton

In order to reach your goal, be prepared to deal with side effects. Some of the most common include fatigue, weakness, headaches, body aches, irritability, insomnia, and depression. Skin problems, such as dryness, itching, and rash frequently occur. So do gastrointestinal complaints, such as nausea, diarrhea, and taste changes. Anemia along with the reduction of platelets and white blood cells are also common.

The question is not if you will have side effects; the question is which ones you will have, how often, how severe, and how you will manage them. Early and aggressive management is a good strategy because it is easier to deal with small problems than to wait for them to become big ones. For instance, a rash in its early stages is much easier to control than one that is so severe that treatment drugs must be stopped.

Throughout the book, I frequently discuss psychiatric problems, especially depression, anxiety, and mania. These side effects are quite common, and usually respond well to medical management. I mention the use of antidepressant medications so often that it may appear that I am pushing their use. Not at all. As a person who only takes medication when absolutely necessary, I too am reluctant to take more pills to combat the side effects of pills. However, psychiatric side effects are the result of chemical changes, which usually respond well to medication. Support, humor, a positive attitude, and the inspiration in this book will provide relief, but they may not be enough if your brain isn't making enough "feel good" chemicals.

Try to keep an open mind about antidepressants, something that I failed to do during my second treatment. I waited far too long, and could have been spared months of low energy because I didn't want to take any more pills. Thoughts of hurting yourself or others may indicate an extreme form of depression and always needs immediate medical attention.

Sources for more information on various side effects are provided under "Side Effects" in the Resources guide at the back of this book.

Don't forget to use the pharmaceutical companies as resources. Contact the company of the medication prescribed for you and ask for free support, information, and tools. You can find the contact information in Resources as well.

I have singled out two side effects—anal/rectal discomfort and rashes. I provide more in-depth detail about how to manage these in Appendices B and C. These side effects tend to occur with telaprevir. Anal/rectal problems are no worse than any other side effect, but are often overlooked and underdiscussed despite being one of the more manageable side effects. I highlight skin problems because they need to be managed proactively. Those taking telaprevir need to be aware of the strong warning for serious skin reactions associated with this medication. Although these reactions are rare, they are potentially fatal. See full prescribing information for a complete warning.

3

●●●●●●●

Readings for the First 12 Weeks

WEEK 1

Day 1

Nothing ventured, nothing gained.

—Proverb

Today you begin what may be the most important endeavor of your life—staking your claim in a future free from hepatitis C. The fear

> **Tip for Today:** Your treatment may likely include self-injection of peginterferon or drugs to manage the side effects. Self-injection can be scary. The instructions may seem daunting. It is normal to worry that you might make a mistake, but it is actually hard to mess it up. Don't worry about injecting air bubbles or hitting a vein. If you are injecting into your belly or thigh with the needle that comes with the medication, it is virtually impossible to hit a vein or damage yourself with an air bubble. Some people get shaky hands when they give themselves the first couple of shots, which is a natural reaction. Take a deep breath and complete the injection when you exhale. You can also try injecting on the count of three. Don't worry too much about your technique. You will have a lot of opportunity to practice and improve.

you have today will pass after you fall into a rhythm with treatment. Just remind yourself of what your goals are and hold fast to this truth: you can do this.

Day 2

Most men have more courage than even they themselves think they have.

—Fulke Greville

It took a lot of courage to start HCV treatment and do that first injection. Treatment may show you that you are stronger and more alive than you ever realized. You can't control your future, but you can shape it.

> **Tip for Today:** Ribavirin needs to be taken with food, and it is better if the food has fat in it. This is also true if you are taking a protease inhibitor, such as boceprevir or telaprevir. The instructions for telaprevir state, *"Eat a meal or snack that contains about 20 grams of fat, within 30 minutes before you take each dose ..."*
>
> This is not a modest amount of fat. You may eat more, but be careful, as weight gain and lipid-related problems may occur. Four eggs or 20 ounces of whole milk yogurt has approximately 20 grams of fat. Nuts are another good source of fat. A list of foods that have approximately 20 grams of fat is provided in Appendix A.

Day 3

Concentrate; put all your eggs in one basket, and watch that basket.

—Andrew Carnegie

In the beginning of treatment, it is easy to stay on track. Your thinking is clear, and your treatment plan is fresh in your mind. This is the best time to establish solid habits, such as using reminders to take your pills. As mentioned in Chapter 2, successful treatment relies on taking your medication as prescribed. You may not be able to control the outcome of your treatment, but you do have control over taking your drugs on time.

Tip for Today: Resolve to find a system that will help you remember to take your medications. A pill container that has three daily compartments is a good investment. You can also use three 7-day pill containers; designate one for morning, afternoon, and evening. If you have trouble devising a foolproof design, ask your medical provider, pharmacist, or drug manufacturer's support line for suggestions.

Day 4

The secret of life is enjoying the passing of time.

—James Thurber

One might argue that another secret to life is regular bowel movements. HCV medications may cause diarrhea and constipation, both associated with the increased fat in your diet. Constipation may also be caused by reduced physical activity or dehydration. If you have loose stools, deal with this problem before it irritates the skin in that region or progresses to diarrhea.

Tip for Today: Talk to your medical provider if you have problems with diarrhea or constipation, particularly if there is a fever, bloody stools, stomach pain, or vomiting. If it is a simple problem, your provider may suggest home remedies. Constipation usually responds to high fiber foods, sufficient liquids, and regular exercise. Diarrhea can be managed by avoiding high fiber or greasy foods. For either diarrhea or constipation, your medical provider may suggest a bulk-forming laxative such as psyllium, which needs to be taken with plenty of water.

Day 5

Every patient carries her or his own doctor inside.

—Albert Schweitzer

We are fortunate to have fantastic medical care along with the real possibility of eliminating HCV and reaping benefits from our efforts. Good medical care is a partnership between a patient and his or her health care team. You are the head of this team, both healer and patient.

Tip for Today: Pharmaceutical companies provide support and information to help HCV patients during treatment. Support includes patient kits, literature, as well as web-based and phone assistance. Find out about available resources by contacting the manufacturer of your HCV medication. Addresses and phone numbers for the pharmaceutical companies that make HCV medications are provided under Resources at the back of this book.

Day 6

Walking is man's best medicine.

—*Hippocrates*

Medicine is more than pills—it is a mind-set. It means learning how to take care of yourself. HCV medications have a better chance of working when we take care of our bodies and minds. There is too much at stake to hope that drugs alone will cure us; we need to participate in the process by giving our bodies an edge, and being fit provides that extra edge.

Tip for Today: If you do not have a regular fitness routine, start one today. Walking has a lot going for it. You can do it anywhere, you don't need expensive equipment, and it is a great way to clear the mind and energize the body. Put on comfortable walking shoes and sunscreen. Step outside and walk 15 minutes or more; then turn around. Make this a daily goal. If 30 minutes is too much, start with whatever you can do. A walk to the mailbox is better than no walk at all. Physical fitness websites are provided in the Resources guide.

Day 7

If we all did the things we are capable of doing, we would literally astound ourselves.

–*Thomas Edison*

Congratulations—you finished your first week of treatment. It is okay to pat yourself on the back; you earned it. Starting treatment is an astounding act of courage. By completing a week of HCV treatment, you have stepped into an elite circle, doing something that many are too afraid to try.

Tip for Today: Do something enjoyable. Life is more than HCV treatment. Read, watch a movie, attend a sporting event, and spend time with friends and family—whatever brings you joy. If you find pleasure in doing nothing, then by all means, do nothing.

WEEK 2

Day 8

Do what you fear and fear disappears.

—*David Schwartz*

Some patients find that the second injection is harder to administer than the first. Although the injections are usually pain-free, there is a psychological component to overcome with self-injection. This is particularly true if you have a history of injection drug use. If you didn't experience any anxiety, appreciate the moment. However, if despite apprehension you went ahead, then you are especially courageous.

Tip for Today: Your skin may still be irritated from your previous injection. This is normal. Some people do not heal for four to six weeks. Rotate your injection sites so that you do not reinject in the same part of your body. If you used your stomach for the first shot, you can use either thigh or the other side of your belly. Report any signs of infection, such as red lines running along your skin, pus, or an area that is swollen or hot when touched. Keep track of your injection sites in your notepad so you can choose a different site next time.

Day 9

The best time to plant a tree was twenty years ago; the second best time is today.

—*Chinese Proverb*

What you do today may affect your health tomorrow. If you want treatment to succeed, take responsibility for your health. For instance, some patients don't commit to a fitness routine because they think they won't feel well during treatment. By now, you have probably figured out that it is possible to maintain good health habits while undergoing treatment. Don't plan on running any marathons, but do plan on finding ways to stay fit.

> **Tip for Today:** HCV treatment is dehydrating. Certain side effects such as fatigue and dryness are easier to manage with adequate water intake. The Institute of Medicine advises that men drink about 13 cups and women consume about 9 cups of liquid daily. If your urine is dark yellow, drink more. It is possible to drink too much water, so don't overdo it. If you can't leave the house because you need to be near a bathroom, then you may be drinking too much.

Day 10

There is no large and difficult task that can't be divided into little easy tasks.

—*Buddhist Proverb*

There is a lot to remember during HCV treatment. Not only do you need to remember to take all of your medications, you also need to store them properly. Put peginterferon in the refrigerator (not the freezer). Ribavirin and telaprevir are stored at room temperature. The manufacturer recommends refrigeration for boceprevir, but it may be stored at room temperature up to 77°F for three months. Keep all medications away from heat.

> **Tip for Today:** Make a checklist of what you need to remember each day, week, and month. Make it a habit to check the list a few times daily, such as each time you eat or turn on your computer, and before bed.

Day 11

Every man is a builder of a temple, called his body, to the god he worships, after a style purely his own, nor can he get off by hammering marble instead. We are all sculptors and painters, and our material is our own flesh and blood and bones.

—*Henry David Thoreau*

By submitting to HCV treatment, you are sculpting your health. You may feel out of sorts or out of control, but there is power in this simple truth—you don't *have* to do treatment, you *get* to do treatment. Take it slowly. You can make it to the end. You will build a magnificent temple.

> **Tip for Today:** Some patients use vitamins, minerals, and herbs to combat HCV treatment side effects, to supplement their diet, and to help with other health issues. Supplements are potent—sometimes they help; sometimes they harm. Do not take St John's wort if you are taking telaprevir or boceprevir. Discuss dietary supplements with your medical provider. More sources for information about supplements are listed under "Complementary and Alternative Medicine" in the Resources at the back of this book.

Day 12

The most beautiful experience we can have is the mysterious.
—Albert Einstein

It is reasonable to fear the unknown. However, great joy can be gained from the unexpected and the mysterious. Sometimes HCV treatment is filled with unanticipated joys. During my own treatment, I learned how kind and generous people are. Try to set aside any fears today and allow for the possibility of an Einstein-like "beautiful experience."

> **Tip for Today:** Although your treatment outcome is unknown, the details of your treatment protocol should not be a mystery. Your medical provider will recommend a schedule for medical visits. By now, your next appointment should be set up, including a scheduled lab test. Maintain a calendar of reminders of medical and lab appointments, prescription renewals, and when to take medication.

Day 13

If one has to submit, it is wasteful not to do so with the best grace possible.
—Winston Churchill

The truth is you don't have to submit to treatment; you made a choice to undergo treatment. You also have a choice to go through this time begrudgingly or with grace. It is likely that your moods will fluctuate—you are human, after all. Mood swings are common during treatment, since the medications affect the brain. However, you can aim for grace and do your best.

Tip for Today: Sufficient sleep is fundamental to health, and it is easier to be graceful when well rested. A good night's sleep and a good mood go hand-in-hand. Strive for seven to nine hours of sleep every night—perhaps more during this time. If you have sleep problems, talk to your medical provider and educate yourself about good sleep habits. Perhaps your sleep is being disturbed by a snoring partner or pet, a problem which is easily fixed with ear plugs. Visit the websites listed in the Resources guide for advice on sleeping smart.

Day 14

I'm not afraid of storms, for I'm learning to sail my ship.
—Louisa May Alcott

Sometimes life feels out of control; other times we feel on top of our game. If aspects of life are overwhelming, look for what you can manage and let go of the rest.

Tip for Today: A common HCV treatment side effect is dry, itchy skin, and this needs to be managed early and aggressively. Start a moisturizing routine, even if you don't notice skin problems, as this may help prevent them. Avoid harsh soaps and use a mild cleanser such as Cetaphil for your body and face. After showering, apply an unscented body cream specifically formulated for sensitive skin. More suggestions are listed in Appendix C: "Managing Skin Problems."

WEEK 3

Day 15

Practice makes perfect.

—Proverb

Most injections aren't painful, but occasionally one may sting or feel downright uncomfortable. The frequency of this usually goes away with practice, as you get better at self-administering injections. Now is a good time to review your technique. Read the instructions again and/or review the video. Instructions are available on the drug manufacturers' websites. Call your pharmacist or medical provider if you have any questions. You can also request an office appointment to review self-injection.

If you are taking oral medication, this is a good time to review your medication management. Are you remembering to take your pills on time?

Tip for Today: If it stings after you self-inject, this may be due to several factors.

- After swabbing your skin, make sure the alcohol has evaporated before you inject.
- Place the bevel of the needle facing up so that the sharpest part enters the skin first.
- Let the medication warm up slightly before administering. Read the manufacturer's instructions on how to safely warm up cold medication or check with your pharmacist or pharmaceutical company.

Day 16

It is in moments of illness that we are compelled to recognize that we live not alone but chained to a creature of a different kingdom, whole worlds apart, who has no knowledge of us and by whom it is impossible to make ourselves understood: our body.

—Marcel Proust

At times, it may feel as if we are alone with our illness, chained to a body and a disease. However, the reality is that there are millions with HCV and hundreds of thousands who have gone through treatment. Take comfort in those numbers—these people who share your disease can help you stay strong.

> **Tip for Today:** Join an HCV group. If you are reluctant because you picture a bunch of people sitting around complaining and crying, think again. HCV groups are fountains of knowledge, laughter, and wisdom. People who share a common disease share a common language and, more importantly, common solutions. Those who have been through treatment ahead of you can tell you what helped, what didn't, and who helped them. There is no better way to invest your time. Besides, it beats staying cooped up at home, feeling sorry for yourself.
>
> To find an HCV support group meeting in your area, visit HCV Advocate at www.hcvadvocate.org and click on Support Groups. For more suggestions on how to find a community or web-based HCV group, see the "Support Groups" section in the Resources guide.

Day 17

An ounce of prevention is worth a pound of cure.

—*Benjamin Franklin*

Right now, your main goal is to take care of yourself and prevent avoidable problems. You and only you are responsible for your body. You may have family, relationships, a job, and other commitments, but for now, make health your priority. If you don't take care of your health, it may be difficult to meet your other responsibilities.

> **Tip for Today:** Don't neglect other health needs while you are treating hepatitis C. Far more people have died from the flu or pneumonia than from HCV. Have you had all the recommended immunizations and are they current? Patients who are undergoing HCV treatment may be immunized during this time. Do not delay this, since vaccines are the best protection against other diseases.

Day 18

Thousands upon thousands of persons have studied disease. Almost no one has studied health.

—Adelle Davis

The time spent during treatment is an opportunity to discover more about health. For instance, you may learn more about lab testing since regular blood tests are an important part of HCV treatment. At first, it may be confusing or overwhelming, but in time, you will understand what is being tested and what those numbers mean.

Tip for Today: Start keeping copies of your medical records. Ask your medical provider for copies of your lab tests and other diagnostic results. Store these in one place. Some people find it helpful to keep a log of results from the most important labs that occur during HCV treatment, such as white blood count (WBCs), hemoglobin (Hgb), platelets, liver enzymes (ALT and AST), and viral load (HCV RNA). If you want more information about lab tests, check out the websites listed in the Resources guide.

Day 19

Commitment is what transforms a promise into reality.

—Abraham Lincoln

Commitment is a radical act. If you are devoted to your health, then it means doing your best to support your goals. Look for aspects of your life that may work against your commitment to health. Choose one small goal that will improve your health.

Tip for Today: Avoiding alcohol is standard advice given by experts to everyone with HCV. This is especially true during HCV treatment. Drinking alcohol during treatment is like applying fertilizer and weed killer simultaneously on weeds and wondering why you still have weeds. If abstaining from alcohol is a problem, get some help. You deserve every chance at successful treatment. If you want more information about alcohol or drug use, see "Substance Use and Recovery" under Resources at the back of this book.

Day 20

A hero is an ordinary individual who finds the strength to persevere and endure in spite of overwhelming obstacles.
—Christopher Reeve

Side effects may be a common occurrence during HCV treatment, but just because they are common doesn't mean that they are acceptable. The trick is to learn how to manage side effects when they are small problems before they become big problems. For instance, if you feel dizzy, that may indicate that you are anemic. If diagnosed early, severe anemia may be avoided by reducing your ribavirin dose. If anemia becomes severe, you may need a blood transfusion or even have to stop taking the HCV medications.

This doesn't mean that you have to call your medical provider the minute you have a side effect. It means that you have to pay attention, and learn when to call your medical provider. Ultimately, it is better to call and find out that a problem isn't a big deal than to err in the other direction. If your doctor has not given you a list of symptoms that need urgent attention, you will find that information in your medication's packaging insert. Chapter 2 provides a list of situations that usually constitute a medical emergency.

Tip for Today: Keep notes or a journal of your questions, issues, and side effects that you want to discuss with your medical provider. Writing things down helps us in a number of ways:
a) It keeps track of what we want to remember;
b) It frees up our minds so we can concentrate on other things;
c) It helps us identify trends or patterns in our treatment.

Day 21

Problems are only opportunities in work clothes.
—Henry Kaiser

One of the myths of HCV treatment is that interferon weakens the immune system. You may feel weaker, but interferon is actually strengthening your immune system. When the immune system is acting properly, it sends interferon to help fight viruses and other microorganisms. When you get a cold, that achy all-over feeling accompanied by the blahs is caused by the body's interferon—not by the actual cold virus. The same is true for the peginterferon you inject for treatment—you are boosting your immune system in order to fight HCV.

Tip for Today: Just because interferon is boosting your immune system, doesn't mean you have to suffer through the symptoms. If you experience body aches and other side effects, talk to your medical provider about how to manage these. Your provider may recommend a nonprescription pain reliever. Some providers recommend alternating between acetaminophen (Tylenol), aspirin, ibuprofen (Advil, Motrin), and naproxen (Naprosyn, Aleve). Follow the instructions on the label and never exceed the recommended dosage. To limit the total dose, check for these ingredients— particularly acetaminophen—in nonprescription and prescription drugs, such as cold and pain medicine (Vicodin, hydrocodone).

WEEK 4

Day 22

One of the things I learned the hard way was that it doesn't pay to get discouraged. Keeping busy and making optimism a way of life can restore your faith in yourself.

—Lucille Ball

Being optimistic is easier said than done; it takes practice and commitment. Keeping busy, especially by helping others, is a good way to keep our heads from listening to a negative feedback loop. It is easier to keep a positive attitude if we surround ourselves with people who tend to be upbeat.

Tip for Today: If you had a one-month supply of HCV medications, make sure you have medication on hand for next week. Call or e-mail today to refill your prescriptions. Set up automatic prescription refills or note in your calendar to call in advance for future refills.

Day 23

When you arise in the morning, think of what a precious privilege it is to think, to enjoy, to love.

—Marcus Aurelius

It may be difficult to appreciate the preciousness of life during treatment, especially when dealing with side effects. If you are battling insomnia and fatigue, you may be understandably moody. Beware—the inability to feel any pleasure may indicate depression, a medical condition best discussed with your medical provider. If you are up to focusing on the precious privileges of life, then hold fast to these sweet moments.

Tip for Today: Headaches make it difficult to think, let alone enjoy life. These common HCV treatment side effects are usually dull, but some people get migraines. Seek medical help if your headaches are severe. Minor headaches usually respond to over-the-counter pain relievers, such as acetaminophen, aspirin, or ibuprofen. However, these medications work best when taken occasionally. Overuse of these drugs may cause a *rebound* headache. A rebound headache occurs when pain relievers wear off and the headache returns.

Day 24

Never deny a diagnosis, but do deny the negative verdict that may go with it.

—Norman Cousins

Norman Cousins, was a remarkable man. He is sometimes described as the "man who laughed his way to health." Cousins used humor to challenge two life-threatening illnesses, and credits Marx Brothers films for helping him manage severe pain. Cousins surrounded himself with humor and brought laughter into the lives of everyone who knew him.

Tip for Today: Make laughter part of your health regimen. Read the comics, watch your favorite comedy show or movie, surf humor websites on the Internet, and attend comedy shows. Consider giving up news and drama while you are on treatment. To stay current, just scan the headlines, but skip any gory details about life's darker side. For more sources of humor, see the Resources at the back of this book.

Day 25

All my possessions for a moment of time.

—Queen Elizabeth I

Patients have an average time of 23 seconds to explain their symptoms before the doctor interrupts them. Given this brief window, prioritize your concerns so that your provider hears the most important issues first. Make eye contact, speak clearly, and starting at the top of your list, use short, clear sentences of what is bothering you the most. For example: "My stomach hurts. I feel nauseous. I have had some diarrhea. I feel tired. I've missed a week of work."

Don't misuse your time this way. "Well, doc, I don't really know if this is something to worry about. It all started last year when I felt a twinge in my right side. I didn't think it was much to worry about, and I didn't want to bother you. Then I felt nauseous …" Your medical provider has a very limited amount of time, and at this point, your conversation will likely be derailed without you having a chance to adequately describe your problem.

> **Tip for Today:** You are probably scheduled to see your medical provider soon. Your appointment will go more smoothly if you prepare for it. If you have been keeping notes about side effects and questions, review and prioritize them. If you haven't kept notes, get organized before the appointment, and jot down any questions or concerns you want to discuss.

Day 26

An individual doesn't get cancer, a family does.

—Terry Tempest Williams

HCV affects more than just us—it touches our families and friends. Those close to you may have fears or concerns about you, your treatment, and your shared future. Communication is essential. Talking and listening to others may help you bypass future problems.

Tip for Today: Ask a family member or friend if he or she wants to go with you to one of your medical appointments or HCV group meetings. This may help family or friends feel more involved, and give them insight into what you may be experiencing. Also, an extra set of ears is a useful tool for keeping accurate medical information. Be sure to tell those who support you how much you appreciate it.

Day 27

Turn your face to the sun and the shadows fall behind you.
—*Maori Proverb*

Maintaining a positive attitude is easier said than done. Surround yourself with light, humor, and positive people. Read inspirational material that reminds you of the positive aspects of life. Go outside and spend time appreciating the world that is illuminated by the sun or a visible moon.

Tip for Today: Sunshine is wonderful, but HCV medications can cause photosensitivity. This is like a sun allergy. You may itch, break out in hives, or burn more easily. Avoid direct sunlight, wear protective clothing, carry an umbrella, and always use sun block. If you do have a sun reaction, apply cool compresses of water or milk to the skin. Your medical provider may suggest an over-the-counter topical cortisone cream or prescribe something to help with sun reactions.

Day 28

The grass must bend when the wind blows across it.
—*Confucius*

You may be noticing more fatigue and other side effects; you may also observe that you are functioning well in spite of being on treatment. This is the perfect time to recommit to your overall health regimen. Ask yourself, what do you need today to stay healthy?

Tip for Today: Good hydration is the cornerstone of side effect management. Make sure you are sipping water throughout the day. Keep a water bottle or glass handy. Store bottled water in an insulated pack in the trunk of the car and out of direct sunlight.

WEEK 5

Day 29

Of course there is no formula for success except perhaps an unconditional acceptance of life and what it brings.
                                                    —*Arthur Rubinstein*

You are beginning your second month of treatment. The injections are probably easier to give. Perhaps you are seeing a pattern with the medication. Some patients notice that they feel more side effects the second or third day after the injection. Others report different patterns. One frustrating aspect of HCV treatment is that it is unpredictable at times and the patterns change. Learn to accept the seemingly random nature of treatment and your journey will be easier.

Tip for Today: If injections are uncomfortable, try this: After cleaning the skin with alcohol, wrap your thumb in a clean tissue and then press firmly on the area for 10 seconds just prior to self-injection; the pressure temporarily confuses the sensory receptors, making it unable to notice sharp sensations. Another tip from patients is to inject after soaking in a hot bath. This may soften the tissue, making it easier to inject.

Day 30

Courage follows action.
                                                    –*Mack R. Douglas*

If you haven't acknowledged your bravery, this is a good time to do so. The hardest part of HCV treatment is deciding to do it; the next hardest part is actually starting it. You are past these monumental feats, so the next challenge is to finish safely. Since you have already proven you are courageous, use this to face future obstacles.

Tip for Today: Workplace disclosure is a concern for patients—should they tell others they are going through HCV treatment? Although there is a certain amount of protection in the workplace, it is impossible to control gossip. Another unfortunate reality is that there is a stigma attached to HCV, particularly because it is potentially infectious. If you have treatment-related mood changes, consider limited disclosure because it provides explanations for behavior changes. People are usually more tolerant when they understand this is a temporary condition. One compromise is to disclose that you are taking a medication for a blood disease and that the medication may alter your mood. If people press for more information you can state that you are uncomfortable discussing it, or give a vague but truthful reply, such as your doctor is treating your immune system.

To learn more about insurance and disability benefits, visit www.hcvadvocate.org and click on the Benefits Column and then HCSP FactSheets to find information about disability, disclosure, and workplace issues.

Day 31

The real voyage of discovery consists not in seeking new landscapes but in having new eyes.

—Marcel Proust

HCV treatment is a voyage of discovery. It is an opportunity to find your own strength and to lean on others. Although treatment is not fun, it is your life's work at this moment. One day you will look back at this time and see how much you have gained, despite the fact that you feel weak.

Tip for Today: Vision and eye problems are common HCV treatment side effects. Most problems are minor, such as dry eyes. If your eyes are extremely dry, or if the natural lubrication gets thick, it may affect your vision. Your medical provider will likely recommend lubricating solution for dry eyes and stronger reading glasses. Of greater concern is retina damage, which could threaten your eyesight. This is rare and nearly always reverses after the medication is discontinued. If you did not have a baseline eye exam before you started taking HCV medications, schedule one today. Always report eye and vision problems to your medical provider.

Day 32

A man too busy to take care of his health is like a mechanic too busy to take care of his tools.
—*Spanish Proverb*

Investing in your health is the best way to avoid illness. Take care of small problems before they become big problems. For instance, a common side effect of telaprevir is anal/rectal discomfort—anal/rectal itching, burning, and hemorrhoids. Initially these may feel like mild annoyances, but if left unattended, they can interfere with the quality of your life.

> **Tip for Today:** One theory about treatment-related anal/rectal burning is that patients may not be absorbing the full dose of telaprevir and that the drug is "leaking out" rather than being fully metabolized. Therefore, not only do patients have anal/rectal discomfort, they are not getting all of their medication. Be sure you are taking all medication as directed; review instructions that accompany your medication. If you are experiencing anal/rectal discomfort, go to Appendix B for ways to manage it.

Day 33

When you come to the end of your rope, tie a knot and hang on.
—*Franklin D. Roosevelt*

HCV medications affect the brain's chemistry, sending patients on an emotional roller coaster. Some of this is normal. However, thoughts of hurting yourself or others is a serious matter needing immediate help. If you have these thoughts, call your medical provider or 911 immediately.

> **Tip for Today:** Antidepressant and anti-anxiety medication can make a huge difference in the quality of one's life. If your doctor suggests trying an antidepressant, don't expect instant results. Some of them take up to six weeks to work. Also, some people need to try several antidepressants to find what is effective and tolerable as these drugs work on different brain pathways. In addition to medication, consider talking to a mental health professional. One can never have too much support. Various resources are listed under "Mental Health" in the Resources guide at the back of this book.

Day 34

Today is only a small manageable segment of time in which our difficulties need not overwhelm us. This lifts from our hearts and minds the heavy weight of both past and future.

—Anonymous

Hepatitis C treatment is best taken one day at a time, with constant medication management. Are you taking all of your drugs on time? This is especially important if you take a direct-acting antiviral, such as telaprevir or boceprevir. If you forget, don't beat yourself up. Don't double up on your medication. Instead, double your efforts to find a plan that will help you remember.

Tip for Today: Here are tricks to help you remember to take your medications on time.

- Use the alarm feature on your cell phone, watch, or computer.
- Wallpaper your world with reminders—use your screen saver or sticky notes.
- Leave voicemail and e-mail reminders to yourself.
- Get an electronic pill reminder.
- If you have a smartphone, use a reminder app.
- Carry extra medication with you in case you don't make it home on time.
- If you live with others, ask them to remind you.
- If you forget a dose, read the guidelines in the literature that accompanies your medication.

Day 35

We are indeed much more than what we eat, but what we eat can nevertheless help us to be much more than what we are.

—Adelle Davis

Every cell in the body relies on good nutrition. We would not expect our cars to run on garbage, yet we expect our bodies to. When we don't eat at regular intervals, it is like expecting our cars to operate without fuel. Make sure that you eat something every three to five hours, depending on your needs.

Tip for Today: Don't skip meals even if you aren't hungry. If lack of appetite is a problem, try small portions consumed more frequently. Sip on smoothies or high-protein shakes. If you feel too tired to prepare food, nibble on toast, cheese, granola, or protein bars. Think outside the box—or inside the box—with a bowl of cereal. For more suggestions, especially for those taking telaprevir, see Appendix A for a list of foods. Also, look at the websites listed under "Nutrition" in Resources at the back of this book.

WEEK 6

Day 36

Prayer is not an old woman's idle amusement. Properly understood and applied, it is the most potent instrument of action.

—Mahatma Gandhi

Scientists and philosophers have long argued about the existence of God and God's ability to heal. I hold that it is a deeply personal issue, one that everyone sorts out individually. Personally, I agree with Gandhi that prayer is a powerful instrument of action. For me, prayer and medicine go hand-in-hand; neither is a substitute for the other, if prayer or a belief in a Higher Power provides strength and comfort, then it seems like a perfect place to turn.

Tip for Today: When times are tough, recite a favorite prayer or phrase. If you don't have spiritual leanings or if you don't have a favorite phrase, try, "This too shall pass." These simple words remind us that HCV treatment is a temporary condition, one that will pass.

Day 37

Be careful about reading health books. You may die of a misprint.

—Mark Twain

The Internet is a powerful resource, but it is also a place of errors, opinions, and advertising. Be critical when collecting information, no matter what the source. Web-based support groups may be helpful, but some participants may sound like experts when they really aren't. People with negative experiences are more likely to voice their opinions than those who have nothing to complain about. If you use the Internet, consider the source and surround yourself with success stories and support.

> **Tip for Today:** Start building your own health library and resources. Include books, websites, and magazine articles. Look for books at garage and library book sales. There are many excellent websites, particularly those run by the government, hospitals, and nonprofit organizations. The Resources guide at the back of this book provides some reliable websites.

Day 38

Visualize winning.

—*Gary Player*

Many successful people believe in the power of visualization. This powerful tool has been used for various health problems, including pain control. If you doubt the power of mind over body, try the following exercise: Close your eyes and relax. Imagine biting into a big, juicy, sour lemon. Notice your reaction. Did you salivate? If so, this illustrates the power of the mind to cause the body to respond to visualization.

> **Tip for Today:** Use visualization on side effects that are interfering with the quality of your life. If you are tired, visualize being alert. If you have insomnia, picture a good night's rest. If you have muscle aches, imagine feeling pain-free. Visualization does not replace medical care, but it can enhance it.

Day 39

If you can't sleep, then get up and do something instead of lying there worrying. It's the worry that gets you, not the lack of sleep.

—*Dale Carnegie*

Insomnia is a common side effect during HCV treatment. One critical element of sleep management is to avoid letting problems become habits. It is harder to change a sleep problem the longer it is established. If you are having sleep difficulties, talk to your medical provider.

Tip for Today: Sleep experts remind us that bedrooms are for sleep and sex—not for tossing and turning. If you lie awake for more than 20 to 30 minutes, get up and do something relaxing, like reading. When you feel tired, go back to bed.

Day 40

Man can live about forty days without food, about three days without water, about eight minutes without air, but only for one second without hope.

—Author Unconfirmed, Attributed to Hal Lindsey

Various religious traditions use 40 days as a benchmark of endurance. Forty days of treatment is certainly noteworthy, and evidence of your strength. Hope, support, and commitment will carry you the rest of the way.

Tip for Today: The 40-day benchmark is a good time to think about your treatment goals and how to stay on course. To reach your goals, use the three R's: Review, remind, and recommit. What were your original goals? Perhaps you chose something simple—to get through treatment. You may have added, "And to do so as easily as possible." Perhaps your goals included remembering to take all of your medication on time. Remind yourself of the reasons why you are undertaking this journey. For many, it is to live free from HCV. Perhaps you are doing this for your family as well as yourself. Are these still your goals? Do you want to modify or add anything? Recommit to the process. You can simply say to yourself, "I am committed to this treatment until the very end." You can formalize your recommitment by writing it down or telling someone your intentions.

Day 41

True courage is like a kite; a contrary wind raises it higher.
—*John Petit-Senn*

Undergoing hepatitis C treatment is an act of courage, particularly when experiencing side effects, such as loss of bone density. While studies looking at the effect of HCV drugs on bone growth have not been conclusive, it is more likely that inactivity is the culprit rather than the drugs themselves. Too much inactivity, particularly excessive bed rest, can lead to bone loss.

Tip for Today: Stay active and strong. Get adequate calcium and vitamin D. The sun is a good source of vitamin D, but between skin cancer and the photosensitivity side effect of HCV medications, supplements are the best way to ensure adequate doses. Also, inadequate vitamin D is associated with poorer HCV treatment results. Talk to your medical provider about the best dose for you.

Day 42

Being deeply loved by someone gives you strength; loving someone deeply gives you courage.
—*Lao Tsu*

Some patients experience sexual difficulties during HCV treatment, such as loss of sex drive, painful intercourse, and erectile dysfunction. These can be frustrating and hard on relationships. Sexual problems may be difficult to talk about, but that is the best way to deal with

Tip for Today: Report sexual problems to your medical provider. Sometimes these are caused by other medications, such as antidepressants. Your provider may want to substitute another antidepressant. If erectile dysfunction is an issue, medications may help, but must be used cautiously with boceprevir and telaprevir. The dosage of erectile dysfunction drugs are usually reduced while on HCV treatment. Ask your medical provider for free samples. Sometimes coupons may be found on the Internet. Women who experience painful intercourse may want to try lubricants, such as K-Y Jelly. Note: If you use a condom or a diaphragm, avoid oil-based lubricants, as these will break down the latex.

this. Try to be open with your sexual partner and explain that this is a common and temporary side effect of HCV medications. Find ways of maintaining intimacy without focusing on sexual intercourse.

WEEK 7

Day 43

Meditation is not a means to an end. It is both the means and the end.
—Jiddu Krishnamurti

Anxiety, irritability, and short-temperedness are common during HCV treatment. Find ways to manage these and not only will you be happier, so will everyone around you. Some patients swear by meditation. The key is to find ways to relax.

> **Tip for Today:** If meditation doesn't interest you, try activities that offer similar benefits. Nature walks, attending a baseball game, bird watching, playing golf, and listening to music can be calming. If you can't manage your mood, talk to your medical provider about this. For more sources of information on meditation, stress reduction, and anger management see the Resources guide at the back of this book.

Day 44

Your pain is the breaking of the shell that encloses your understanding.
—Kahlil Gibran

For most, good side effect management makes a huge difference in the quality of HCV treatment. This doesn't necessarily mean taking more pills in order to stay on your medication. In addition to discussing

> **Tip for Today:** The hardest side effect for me to deal with was relentless nausea. It can be alleviated by eating fresh ginger, drinking peppermint or raspberry leaf tea, or pressing the acupressure points on the wrists. Since hunger can intensify nausea, try eating a bit of food every hour, such as a cracker. Your doctor may prescribe something for you or suggest an over-the-counter drug.

side effect management with your medical provider, spend some time researching nonprescription ways to cope with your side effects.

Day 45

The mind grows sicker than the body in contemplation of its suffering.
—Ovid

Living with HCV and its treatment is an exercise in balance. Sometimes it is relatively easy and doesn't require much thought; other times it can feel like walking a tightrope. Regardless, it helps not to dwell on it. Thinking too much about HCV and how bad you feel at this moment in time, can add a layer of suffering that can make treatment feel unbearable.

> **Tip for Today:** Develop a support system of people you can talk to when times get tough. Sometimes it is better to talk to people outside of your immediate family. In particular, find people who are willing to listen without judging you and who will give you honest advice if you ask for it. Even better, develop relationships with people who have been through HCV treatment and have some idea of what you are going through.

Day 46

A violent wind does not outlast the morning; a squall of rain does not outlast the day. Such is the course of Nature. And if Nature herself cannot sustain her efforts long, how much less can man!
—Lao Tzu

Nature may feel like an obstacle in life, particularly the nature in our own bodies. You may occasionally feel light-headed or dizzy. Although

> **Tip for Today:** Lightheadedness during treatment can be caused by various factors, such as anemia, low blood pressure, and dehydration. Your medical provider will rule out medical causes. Make sure that you are drinking plenty of liquids and are eating at regular intervals. After sitting or lying down, get up slowly. Pump blood to your upper body by squeezing the muscles in your legs and hips as you stand up.

you need to report this and other side effects to your medical provider, light-headedness is common and usually not cause for panic. Fear and anxiety may intensify the problem. When we get scared, we hold our breath or breathe shallowly. Lightheadedness is a time for more oxygen, not less. If this happens, breathe deeply and slowly. If you feel lightheaded, sit or lie down and tell someone you feel faint.

Day 47

I never worry about action, but only inaction.
—*Winston Churchill*

Sometimes patients are reluctant to get help for side effects. They think, "Maybe this will go away," or "I'll wait until my next appointment." These are reasonable responses, but don't wait too long. A small problem is easier to fix than a big one.

> **Tip for Today:** An effective tool to consider is the pharmaceutical companies' patient support resources. These are free and include a phone line where you can talk to nurses. It helps to have many tools at our disposal.

Day 48

A successful person is one who can lay a firm foundation with the bricks that others throw at him.
—*David Brinkley*

Sometimes it feels like life is throwing bricks at us, and bricks can feel especially heavy during this time. Take it easy and deal with one brick at a time. You are building a firm foundation of health.

> **Tip for Today:** A frustrating aspect of treatment is it seems unpredictable. Some days are harder than others are. If you have a difficult day, it can be tempting to worry that all future days will be hard, or to think, "If today is this tough, then how much harder will it be a month or more from now?" However, treatment doesn't act like that. It isn't a straight line. This unpredictable course is challenging. Take it brick by brick.

Day 49

If you want to feel rich, just count the things you have that money can't buy.

—*Proverb*

HCV treatment is expensive and by now, you know what your monthly cost is for the drugs. However, if you are having side effects, you may encounter more costs, particularly for other injectable drugs, such as those that stimulate blood cell production. Remind yourself that your health is your real measurement of wealth, and you are investing in your future.

Tip for Today: Explore options to ease the financial burden of drug costs. A useful resource is *Needy Meds* www.needymeds.com. This provides discounts, coupons, and financial help to nearly everyone, including assistance for buying prescription drugs for pets. This website is extensive and constantly updating, so don't just look at it once. For more, go to the "Financial Issues and Medical Insurance" section in the Resources guide at the back of this book.

WEEK 8

Day 50

Never, never, never, never give up.

—*Winston Churchill*

Every time you give yourself an injection or take your pills, you are honoring your commitment to your health. You may feel like quitting at times, but remember that your life is in your hands. If you feel like giving up, review your goals, talk to a friend, or call your medical provider. Extra support or help with side effects may help you get through temporary obstacles.

Tip for Today: Make sure you refill your prescriptions. If you are due for lab tests or medical appointments, be sure to follow-up on these. You can set up reminders on your cellular phone, computer, or calendar.

Day 51

Think of all the beauty still left around you and be happy.
—Anne Frank

We all know that "beauty is only skin deep" and "beauty is in the eye of the beholder." No matter how much we believe these things, it is natural to want to look our best. At the same time, you may be feeling tired and not wanting to spend much time fussing over your appearance. This is a good time to find shortcuts and keep things simple.

Tip for Today: Don't neglect yourself—when we look good, we feel good. You may have heard that you shouldn't use harsh chemicals on your hair during treatment. This is because HCV medications dry out the hair and leave it brittle. However, you can still color your hair, especially if you use a gentler product, such as semi-permanent hair color. Unlike harsher permanent colors, semi-permanent ones are gentler because they don't penetrate the hair shaft as deeply. You may have to color your hair more often but you don't have to give it up altogether. Alternatively, you may want to seize the opportunity to go natural.

Day 52

The fishermen know that the sea is dangerous and the storm terrible, but they have never found those dangers sufficient reason for remaining ashore.
—Vincent van Gogh

Sometimes HCV treatment feels like drowning in an ocean of side effects, particularly if plagued by fatigue. Many factors can contribute to fatigue—low thyroid, insomnia, and diabetes, to name a few. Ribavirin causes hemolytic anemia, which will leave one feeling quite tired.

Tip for Today: Hemolytic anemia is common and can be managed if caught early. Regular lab tests are essential. If ignored, this form of anemia is serious and could threaten your life and ability to stay on treatment. This type of anemia has nothing to do with low iron. Excess iron can cause liver damage and should never be taken unless prescribed.

The medication causes the red blood cells to burst, leaving the body with insufficient oxygen-carrying capacity. It's like running a car on two or three cylinders.

Day 53

It's so hard when I have to, and so easy when I want to.

—*Sondra Anice Barnes*

When you feel low or resistant to treatment, try to identify the cause. Perhaps side effects are bothering you. Have you talked to your medical provider about these? If you have, but you still have problems, do you need to wait until the remedy kicks in? Maybe you are too accommodating and need to be more persistent in seeking solutions. If you haven't reported your problems to your medical provider, is this because you are afraid that your treatment will be stopped? This is unlikely. In fact, you are better off addressing problems in the early stages when they are small, rather than letting the problems get bigger and harder to fix.

Tip for Today: By now, you are probably seeing that sometimes treatment is hard. Feeling sorry for yourself is normal. Try improving your mood by saying, *I don't have to do treatment— I get to do treatment.* If you are feeling low because of medication side effects, call your medical provider and get some help with this.

Day 54

Listen to what you know instead of what you fear.

—*Richard Bach*

If you haven't already had an abnormal lab result, you will eventually. This is so common that it is expected. Try not to react with fear over an abnormal result. This will help keep your head clear so that you can learn more facts about your condition. Fear doesn't help anybody and it can feel downright miserable.

Tip for Today: HCV medications usually cause abnormal lab tests, especially to the various components of the complete blood count (CBC). Typically, white blood cells drop dramatically; so do platelets and red blood cells. However, just because they are abnormal doesn't mean you are sick. There is a range of abnormal results that is perfectly acceptable. To a certain extent, most of us can tolerate a substantial drop in white cells and platelets. Red blood cells are trickier because if they drop too low this lowers your hemoglobin, which carries oxygen to all the cells in your body. If your hemoglobin gets too low, your medical provider may reduce your ribavirin or suggest using another injectable drug that stimulates red blood cell production. Never judge your labs by a single result; instead look for trends.

Day 55

I seldom think about my limitations, and they never make me sad. Perhaps there is just a touch of yearning at times; but it is vague, like a breeze among flowers.

—*Helen Keller*

HCV treatment may cause problems with concentration, memory, and foggy thinking. This can be very frustrating, particularly since we need to rely on our brains to help us remember to take medication, to work, to learn, and to function. Frustration drains us of valuable resources because we are by focusing on problems. Let go of frustration and your brain is free to find solutions.

Tip for Today: Focus on what is working rather than what isn't working. If concentration is less than perfect, look at the bigger picture. Can you see situations where things could be worse? Remind yourself of the temporary nature of this situation. Entertain the possibility that your life might improve at any moment. Concentration may improve with brain games; look for websites under the "Brain Fitness" section in the Resources guide.

Day 56

Yoga teaches us to cure what need not be endured and endure what cannot be cured.

—B.K.S. Iyengar

Regular physical activity is one of the most effective weapons against HCV treatment's side effects. Interferon causes aches, pains, and stiffness, which can become worse when you slow down and reduce your physical activity. Stay as active as possible. Yoga, Pilates, tai chi, qigong, stretching, walking, gardening, and dancing are excellent ways to remain active, flexible, and in condition.

> **Tip for Today:** There are many ways to incorporate physical fitness into our lives. Look for classes in your community. Check out videos or books from your library. The Internet provides a wealth of fitness information. YouTube has a great selection of fitness videos. You can exercise and stretch while watching TV. If you have a stationary bike or treadmill, use it. You can strengthen your muscles with light weights or exercise bands. If you don't own hand weights, filled water bottles or soup cans are good substitutes.

WEEK 9

Day 57

As far as inner transformation is concerned, there is nothing you can do about it. You cannot transform yourself, and you certainly cannot transform your partner or anybody else. All you can do is create a space for transformation to happen, for grace and love to enter.

—Eckhart Tolle

You cannot control the outcome of this treatment, but you can try to control your attitude. How do you feel about taking medications, particularly one that is self-injected? Do you view the drugs as poison or as medicine? When we focus on the positive, we activate neurochemicals in our brains that can help us in all sorts of ways, such as by boosting the immune system and cognitive ability. Focusing on the negative just produces more negativity.

> **Tip for Today:** Create a space for transformation. This can be an actual place or visualized in your mind. On injection days, instead of viewing the procedure as cold and clinical, welcome the medication and the tools you use to administer it. Invite the process; transform it into a ritual of healing.

Day 58

Water is life's mater and matrix, mother and medium. There is no life without water.

—*Albert Szent-Györgyi*

Most patients complain of nearly constant dry mouth problems. Some days it may feel like you are stranded in a desert. Drinking liquids is the best remedy for this. Remind yourself that, like most side effects, dryness is temporary.

> **Tip for Today:** Sip water through the day. Suck on ice chips, sugar-free candy, or gum. Try dental products specifically formulated for dry mouths. Look for these at your drugstore or talk to your dentist.

Day 59

Happiness is having a scratch for every itch.

—*Ogden Nash*

Happiness is having no itch to scratch. Unfortunately, itching happens, and it is particularly maddening when the itch is in the anal

> **Tip for Today:** The main points to remember about anal/rectal discomfort are:
> - Be sure you are taking your medication with high-fat food.
> - If you have diarrhea or loose stools, ask your medical provider for help to get it under control.
> - Keep the anal area clean and dry.
> - Protect the skin on your bottom.
> - More on managing of anal/rectal discomfort is provided in Appendix B.

region. In addition to itching, there can be burning or pain. This awful side effect has a hitch to it—it isn't something that is mentioned in public. The only people who understand the seriousness of this are patients who have HCV treatment experience, and, hopefully, your medical provider.

Day 60

Commitment is an act, not a word.

—Jean-Paul Sartre

Although you may be feeling side effects from the HCV medications, some days you are probably feeling better than you thought you would. Perhaps flu-like symptoms occur occasionally, but it is unlikely that these interfere with your routine. This is a good time to commit to your overall health goals—physical, emotional, and spiritual.

> **Tip for Today:** Commitment means taking care of your entire body, including your mouth. Treatment can be hard on the teeth and gums. This is a good time to perform good dental hygiene. Make sure you schedule regular dental cleanings and check-ups. If you aren't already accustomed to daily flossing, this is a good time to start. The hardest part of establishing a new habit is remembering to do it. Leave the floss out on the bathroom counter or other place where you can see it. If you watch TV in the evenings, put the floss where you sit as a reminder to use it.

Day 61

When written in Chinese, the word "crisis" is composed of two characters. One represents danger and the other represents opportunity.

—John F. Kennedy

HCV treatment is different for everyone. The side effects and their intensity vary, and people manage them in different ways. Some patients ignore them and hope they go away, while others notice side effects immediately. Patients may be afraid that if they don't deal with a problem immediately that it will get worse. A few problems need immediate attention, such as chest pain, a high fever, or thoughts of suicide. Most problems can wait until your medical provider's regular office hours.

Tip for Today: It helps to know the difference between emergency problems, problems that aren't urgent but need prompt attention, and conditions that can wait until your next medical appointment. Perhaps your medical provider gave you instructions on when to call the office or 911. Chest pain, breathing difficulties, and thoughts of harming yourself or others require immediate care. Also urgent are weakness, loss of coordination, numbness, or difficulty speaking. If you aren't sure of the seriousness of a problem, it's better to call and let your provider make the decision. Eventually you will get a sense of how quickly to seek medical attention.

Day 62

Do not betray me! Work on! Do not arrest my song.
—Pablo Neruda, Translated by Oriana Kalant

With more than 500 functions, the liver is the body's workhorse. Your liver is constantly making new cells, especially now that it has a break from HCV's constant assault. This organ is so amazing that Pablo Neruda wrote a poem about it, *Oda al Hígado.*

Tip for Today: Everything goes through the liver. Avoid chemicals, fumes, alcohol, certain drugs and dietary supplements, raw or undercooked shellfish, and wild foraged mushrooms. Think before you put it into your mouth, breathe it, or apply it to your body.

Day 63

Gratitude can turn a meal into a feast, a house into a home, a stranger into a friend. It makes sense of our past, brings peace for today, and creates a vision for tomorrow.
—Melody Beattie

I used to roll my eyes when people said the secret to life is living in gratitude. I thought you had to have something to be thankful for in order to express gratitude. Now I know that simply being alive is plenty to be grateful for, and when I appreciate this, life is easier.

Tip for Today: Make a gratitude list. Do this even if your heart isn't in to it. It's amazing what happens to us when we appreciate even the littlest things.

WEEK 10

Day 64

We are given one life, and the decision is ours whether to wait for circumstances to make up our mind, or whether to act, and in acting, to live.

—Omar Nelson Bradley

You are now starting your 10th week, measuring your progress in double digits. You made a decision to take your future into your own hands. You followed through on your treatment and you are still hanging in there. You are amazing!

Tip for Today: Take a moment to look at other aspects of your health that may need attention. Are you exercising, drinking sufficient liquids, eating well, and sleeping enough? Do you have any HCV treatment side effects that are weighing on you that may need medical intervention? Don't let side effects and other medical issues get out of control. For more tips on how to manage side effects, look at the websites listed in the Resources guide.

Day 65

Hold on; hold fast; hold out. Patience is genius.
—Georges-Louis Leclerc, Comte de Buffon

Patience is not just sitting around, gritting your teeth, and wallowing in agony. Patience is action. It is the art of waiting for a solution when you least feel like waiting, while having faith that you will get through this difficulty.

Tip for Today: Patience is a tool that patients can use to help endure side effects, such as a chronic cough. This common HCV treatment side effect is generally not a big deal, but since a cough could be the symptom of something more serious, report it to your medical provider. Prescription or over-the-counter cough medication may help. Drink plenty of liquids, suck on cough drops or sugarless lozenges, and use steam or a humidifier to soothe your mucous membranes. Add a dose of patience to your recovery plan.

Day 66

Think not, is my eleventh commandment, and sleep when you can, is my twelfth.
—*Herman Melville*

Sleep is a basic function. So much depends on sufficient sleep. Our moods, health, and ability to enjoy life are all affected with this activity. If you are bothered by insomnia, don't let it continue any longer. Talk to your medical provider. Learn about sleep hygiene on the Internet or at your library.

Tip for Today: Turn your bedroom into a place that promotes sleep. The room should be dark, quiet, and cool. If noise is a problem, try earplugs. Wax or silicone earplugs are especially effective. Keep TV out of the bedroom. If you find yourself thinking instead of sleeping, try listening to relaxing music, audio books, or podcasts.

Day 67

When life's problems seem overwhelming, look around and see what other people are coping with. You may consider yourself fortunate.
—*Ann Landers*

Some HCV side effects are hard to deal with and it is easy to start feeling sorry for oneself. Mouth sores are a good example. A bad case of these makes it hard to eat, and the pain is difficult to manage. There are some home remedies for mouth sores, but some cases are so painful that medical intervention is necessary.

> **Tip for Today:** Talk to your medical provider if you develop mouth pain or sores. Avoid foods that are hard, crunchy, spicy, salty, or acidic. Do not drink excessively hot liquids. Ice or frozen juice bars may soothe mouth pain. Try over-the-counter products that numb canker sores or apply a protective barrier to lesions. Your dentist may be able to recommend a prescription rinse to help.

Day 68

It's not the work which kills people, it's the worry. It's not the revolution that destroys machinery, it's the friction.

—Henry Ward Beecher

Friction and resistance can make everything seem harder. Sometimes it is best to go with the flow. If you are feeling achy, perhaps this is worse because you are carrying tension in your muscles. Try to pay attention to the stress you carry and find ways to let it go.

> **Tip for Today:** Muscle and joint pain respond well to gentle movement. Avoid long periods of inactivity. For minor body aches, try heating pads, ice packs, hot baths, massage, stretching, walking, tai chi, Pilates, or yoga.

Day 69

I teach my sighs to lengthen into songs.

—Theodore Roethke

Chronic HCV infection is odd in so many ways. It isn't an urgent condition, like a heart attack. Some people don't have symptoms of the disease, such as a tumor, giving them signals that something is wrong. Yet even those without cirrhosis submit to this long and difficult treatment anyway, uncertain of how much damage HCV will do. Treatment provides opportunities to turn sighs into songs.

Tip for Today: Here is something to sing about—caffeine. There have been a number of studies about coffee and HCV. Coffee drinkers have lower risk of fibrosis and cirrhosis. Coffee drinkers are more like to respond to HCV treatment and tolerate side effects better. However, caffeine may interfere with sleep, so drink your coffee early in the day.

Day 70

Patience is not passive. On the contrary, it is active; it is concentrated strength.

—*Edward G. Bulwer-Lytton*

In the beginning, it may seem like a long time until the end of HCV treatment. Many patients say that initially, treatment is always on their mind. After a while, if the side effects aren't too bad, it becomes just another part of life. However, sometimes a side effect will be so uncomfortable that it takes a lot of effort to remain committed. If this happens, make sure you talk to your medical provider and your support system.

Tip for Today: Itching can wear the patience of saints, but try to avoid scratching. The best way to manage dry, itchy skin is to prevent it. Apply fragrance-free, hypoallergenic creams immediately following bathing. Creams are generally more effective than lotions. Add a couple of drops of lightweight oil to cream for extra protection. Medication may be the best way to control itching; discuss this with your medical provider.

WEEK 11

Day 71

Hope doesn't come from calculating whether the good news is winning out over the bad. It's simply a choice to take action.

—*Anna Lappé*

Each time you take care of yourself you step into action. When you take your medication, get enough sleep, eat something nutritious, or call your doctor, you demonstrate the power of hope.

Tip for Today: Supplement the power of hope with the power of action. Take control by avoiding colds and viruses. Hand washing is one of the best ways to protect yourself from unwanted illnesses. Effective hand washing needs to be done for 20 to 30 seconds—about the time it takes to sing the alphabet song, twice if you are a fast singer. In public places, sing it silently if you want to avoid strange looks from others. If you want more information about how to take better care of yourself, the Resources' "General Health" section lists some excellent websites.

Day 72

Misery is a communicable disease.

—Martha Graham

Although misery is contagious, so is joy. If you are around negative people who seem to bring you down, pursue relationships with those who make you feel better.

Tip for Today: If your viral load results are undetectable for HCV, you may wonder if you still have a communicable disease. A good practice is for everyone always to treat blood as if it is potentially infectious; this protects you and others. Don't share any personal hygiene articles that may come into contact with blood, such as razors, toothbrushes, or cuticle scissors. Cover cuts and wounds and safely dispose of sanitary products. Clean up blood spills with household bleach (1 part bleach to 10 parts water). Check out the Resources guide for more about HCV transmission.

Day 73

I have learned never to underestimate the healing power we all have. It is always there to be used for the highest good. We just have to remember to use it.

—Mark Victor Hansen

Sometimes you may feel swept away by side effects and lose track that your body is trying to heal itself. Bear in mind that the point of taking antiviral medications is to reach a new level of healing and quite possibly rid your body of HCV. Your body's natural inclination is to heal. Don't let your head get in the way of this.

> **Tip for Today:** Use caution if you take dietary supplements to manage your health, especially since these may interact with any drugs you are taking. For instance, if you are anemic from ribavirin, you may be tempted to take iron. However, iron won't fix ribavirin-induced anemia unless your iron levels are low, and taking it without medical advice can be dangerous for your liver. Herbs and other dietary supplements may be helpful when used appropriately; it's best to use these under expert guidance. Do not take St John's wort if you are taking an HCV or HIV protease inhibitor.

Day 74

Laughter is inner jogging.

—*Norman Cousins*

Science has studied the health benefits of humor. It boosts the immune system, reduces pain, and has numerous other benefits. It is free, painless, requires little commitment, and is fun. Even better, it doesn't require a prescription. If your spirit is waning, order humor for yourself today.

> **Tip for Today:** Find ways to bring more laughter into your life. Some easy suggestions are to get a joke-a-day on the Internet, download humorous podcasts, watch reruns of favorite comedy programs, or check out old comedy radio shows from the library.

Day 75

Finish each day and be done with it. You have done what you could. Some blunders and absurdities no doubt crept in; forget them as soon as you can. Tomorrow is a new day; begin it well and serenely and with too high a spirit to be encumbered with your old nonsense.

—*Ralph Waldo Emerson*

It is all too easy to get stuck in our heads—to be running the same thoughts over and over. Some of this may be from the HCV medications; some from living with fatigue and other side effects; some from being human. Try to develop ways to shake off a negative inner voice and to start with a clean slate every day.

Tip for Today: Sometimes stuck thoughts are actually symptoms of the neuropsychiatric side effects of HCV medications. If you find yourself feeling overwhelmed and hassled by your thought process, tell your medical provider. Better yet, ask for a referral to a psychiatrist who understands the side effects of HCV treatment. If your symptoms are caused by HCV medications, psychiatric medications are wonderful when they work and may provide relief as you go through treatment.

Day 76

Shoot for the moon. Even if you miss, you will land in the stars.

—Les Brown

One common concern is that HCV treatment will interfere with employment. By now, you probably have a sense of your capacity to work. Continuing to work during treatment has its advantages. In addition to maintaining your income, it is a great distraction.

Tip for Today: Try to keep your life simple. If you are working, don't take on too much outside of work. Find ways to rest; take breaks. Delegate, take shortcuts, ask for help, and lower your standards. You don't have to do everything just as you would have done it before treatment or perfectly.

- Request a change in responsibility. Perhaps you have a project that demands too much of you and work would be easier if you did not have this one responsibility.
- Take breaks. Perhaps you can take a nap in the employee lounge or in your car, with the doors locked and parked in a safe place.
- Explore creative ways to lighten your load, such as job sharing, working from home, or using sick leave to reduce work hours.

HCV side effects are bad enough, but if you don't have anything to do but to think about them, side effects can magnify. Naturally, if treatment interferes with your work, then talk to your medical provider about this. If medical leave is best for your situation, then by all means, do it.

Day 77

Healing, Papa would tell me, is not a science, but the intuitive art of wooing Nature.

—W. H. Auden

Nature soothes mind, body, and spirit. If you are feeling cooped up by work, personal obligations, and HCV treatment, you may need a break. Nature is all around us—we just have to see and feel it. If weather conditions are harsh, nature can be enjoyed from inside.

Tip for Today: Pursue opportunities to be around nature. Go for a walk, rest on a park bench, or drive to a favorite quiet spot. Sit by a window and enjoy a cup of tea. Put fresh flowers or a plant near where you spend most of your day. Keep a seashell, rock, or photo to remind you of nature's beauty.

WEEK 12

Day 78

Nothing in life is to be feared. It is only to be understood.

—Marie Curie

Soon you will have your week 12 labs done. If for some reason no labs have been ordered, talk to your medical provider. If your results are abnormal, don't panic. It is normal to have abnormal labs during HCV treatment. The issue is not *if* so much as *how abnormal*? Someone on the medical staff should explain the results to you and give you a copy.

Tip for Today: Never let a lab result dictate how you are feeling. If you don't feel well and your lab results are normal, don't dismiss your feelings. If you feel well and your lab results are abnormal, try not to scare yourself into feeling sick. Some labs, such as your white blood count, may be abnormally low but no symptoms are associated with this, so you won't feel it. Also, if you are feeling poorly and your lab results are abnormal, that doesn't mean that the cause is related to the labs. For instance, you may feel fatigued and if your hemoglobin is low, that would explain it. However, you may also be experiencing depression or insomnia. If these are contributing and addressed, you may feel less tired.

Day 79

Love does not begin and end the way we seem to think it does. Love is a battle, love is a war; love is a growing up.

—*James Baldwin*

While I was on treatment, the arguments I had with my husband were ridiculous. I was childish, acting in ways I would not normally. After treatment was over and I returned to my normal self, I had some apologies to make. What I didn't realize was how powerless my husband felt.

Tip for Today: If your community offers a support group for caregivers, ask those in your life who are affected by your treatment if they will attend. If you know the family or friends of anyone who has gone through treatment, perhaps they would be willing to talk to those in your relationship circle.

Day 80

A man without a goal is like a ship without a rudder.

—*Thomas Carlyle*

Another forty days have passed. This means you have completed two back-to-back journeys into a wilderness of side effects. You may not see how strong and amazing you are, but you are.

> **Tip for Today:** This is a good time to go over the three R's: Review, Remind, and Recommit. Review your goals. Remind yourself of the reasons why you are undertaking this journey. Recommit to the process. Then tell yourself how strong and amazing you are.

Day 81

Thoughts are like birds flying overhead—you can't control them—but you certainly can stop them from making a nest in your hair.
—Buddhist Proverb

Few have endured HCV treatment without some difficulty, and thinking about your challenges is inevitable. These moments pass. The trick is to refrain from making these moments worse by focusing on them.

> **Tip for Today:** Picture your negative thoughts as if they are birds flying overhead. If you are thinking about something too much, imagine it flying away. If the thoughts won't go way, write down on a piece of paper what is bothering you, and put it in a box on a shelf. Take the piece of paper out of the box once a day and think about it all you want. Then put it back in the box. If you start ruminating again, remind yourself that the thought is in the box and you can think about it later when you open the box. Invite positive thoughts to build nests in your head.

Day 82

I'm tired of all this nonsense about beauty being only skin-deep. That's deep enough. What do you want, an adorable pancreas?
—Jean Kerr

Let's face it, HCV treatment is not exactly a beauty treatment. Granted, beauty is less important than your health, but many of us get a lift when we look our best. A side effect that may be noticeable soon, if it hasn't already started, is hair loss. Don't despair. This is a temporary situation, and one that can be minimized with various remedies. While you are experimenting with ways to appear more attractive, keep in mind that your liver probably looks better than it has in a long time.

> **Tip for Today:** If your hair is thin or dull, try hair products that work with these limitations. If you color or curl your hair, reduce the frequency and use the mildest chemicals possible. Vegetable-based hair color is a gentler choice. A professional hair stylist may suggest a style or products that will add body and shine to your hair.

Day 83

The secret of health for both mind and body is not to mourn for the past, worry about the future, or anticipate troubles, but to live in the present moment wisely and earnestly.

—Buddha

We might find ourselves worrying even on our best days. Yet, isn't worrying a bit like paying mortgage on a house we might buy but don't live in yet? Today is a good day to try living in the present.

> **Tip for Today:** There are many ways to quiet the mind and to live in the moment. Here is one to try: Sitting or lying down, inhale slowly and deeply into your abdomen as if it was a balloon. Imagine you are breathing in peace, filling your entire body with it. Notice and relax any tension in your body, breathing into those areas. Exhale deeply, ridding yourself of worry. Practice this throughout the day.

Day 84

The journey is the reward.

—Chinese Proverb

Congratulations. You made it through the first 12 weeks of treatment. For those of you with genotype 2 or 3, or for other genotypes who meet the criteria of response-guided therapy, this is usually the halfway point. If you made it this far, you can make it the rest of the way, and you are very likely to eradicate HCV permanently. Skip to Chapter 6, "Readings for the Final 12 Weeks." If you do not know the length of your treatment yet, continue with the next chapter. You can skip ahead if your treatment length is shortened to 24 weeks.

For those on a 28-week treatment plan, you are almost at your halfway mark. You are a mere two weeks from this milestone.

For others, it marks completion of the first quarter. You now know what to expect during treatment. It is unlikely to get harder, although there may be a few bumps ahead. Just hang on. If you made it this far, you can make it all the way. I know this through my own 48-week treatment, and having walked with many others through theirs. Continue reading with the next chapter.

A small fraction of you may be stopping treatment at this point either because of medical reasons, or because your treatment plan was only for twelve weeks. If it was because you are done, sit back and enjoy your recovery. You will be feeling much better in a few weeks.

If you are stopping treatment because of medical reasons, these words are for you: Whether you are stopping because the medications aren't working, or because of unmanageable side effects, do not drown in disappointment or regret. Although you did not have the outcome you wanted, your liver benefited from even a short stint of treatment. Some patients never even try treatment, and you gave it your best. You fought hard, and in my book, that makes you a winner. The information in Chapter 8, "When Treatment Doesn't Work," will help you through your next phase.

Tip for Today: Celebrate your success of making it through 12 weeks of HCV treatment. You accomplished something that others will never even try. Do something special for yourself to honor the distance you have travelled.

4

●●●●●○○

Readings for Weeks 13 through 24

If at any point you are discontinuing treatment because the medications are not working or side effects force you to quit, skip to Chapter 8, "When Treatment Doesn't Work." If you discontinue early but don't know the results yet, you can read Chapter 7, "Waiting for Results."

WEEK 13

Day 85

It's also helpful to realize that this very body that we have, that's sitting right here right now ... with its aches and its pleasures ... is exactly what we need to be fully human, fully awake, fully alive.

—Pema Chödrön

At this point, you may have more aches than pleasures and be unlikely to find much comfort in these words. It may be more accurate to describe yourself as fully human, fully exhausted, and fully irritated. If this is how you are feeling, you are fully into HCV treatment.

Tip for Today: One of the worst side effects is nausea. If you are plagued with this, try tips recommended for motion sickness, morning sickness, or chemotherapy-induced nausea. Many products alleviate nausea, such as Preggie Pops or Queasy Drops/Pops. Ginger is helpful and comes in multiple forms—fresh, candied, ginger drops, or ginger tea. Chamomile or raspberry leaf tea may also soothe the stomach.

Day 86

When the bridge is gone, the narrowest plank becomes precious.
—Hungarian Proverb

Complementary and alternative medicine (CAM) may provide a bridge between tolerable side effects and intolerable ones. CAM is more than herbs and supplements; it includes a variety of healing arts, such as acupuncture, ayurveda, hypnotherapy, massage therapy, and other bodywork. Some insurance companies cover CAM if a physician refers you.

Tip for Today: You can apply self-help methods, such as qigong exercises. *The Hepatitis C Help Book* by Misha Ruth Cohen and Robert Gish is written specifically for those with HCV and provides some self-help techniques. A self-help acupressure factsheet can be found at www.hcvadvocate.org.

Day 87

Each morning when I open my eyes I say to myself: I, not events, have the power to make me happy or unhappy today. I can choose which it shall be. Yesterday is dead, tomorrow hasn't arrived yet. I have just one day, today, and I'm going to be happy in it.
—Groucho Marx

HCV medications affect our moods. Although this is a physiological reaction, that doesn't mean that we are completely powerless. Our thoughts can also influence our disposition. Use the power of positive thinking to give you an edge against moodiness.

> **Tip for Today:** Try pushing yourself beyond your comfort zone. Get out of bed, stand tall, and get out of the house. Engage in activity that used to bring pleasure—go to a movie, visit friends, and walk in a park. Pursue pleasure with a delightful vengeance.

Day 88

Laughter and tears are both responses to frustration and exhaustion. I myself prefer to laugh, since there is less cleaning up to do afterward.
—*Kurt Vonnegut*

I did all sorts of silly things during treatment. I posted a note on my dashboard reminding me to get gas. However, I placed it over the gas gauge and didn't see the low fuel light go on, so I ran out of gas. I can laugh at it now, but at the time, I couldn't decide who I should call first—the auto club or the crisis hotline.

> **Tip for Today:** There may be times when you aren't able to laugh at yourself no matter how hard you try. Apply damage control by not making things worse than they are. If stress or anger management is a problem, talk to your medical provider, as these may be medication-induced. It may help to learn a few simple techniques to manage these symptoms.

Day 89

Laugh at yourself first, before anyone else can.
—*Elsa Maxwell*

A common phenomenon in HCV treatment is that you usually look better than you feel. The weird thing is that patients sometimes complain about this. They want people to know that they don't feel well. Patients don't want to have to explain that they feel horrible, and they certainly don't want people to think they are lying about how they feel, just because they look halfway decent.

Tip for Today: Accept that you probably look better than you feel. Don't expect others to be able to guess how you feel. If you are concerned that others will think you are capable of more than you feel up to, be honest about it. While you are at it, laugh at yourself. Isn't it kind of silly to be annoyed that you don't look half bad?

Day 90

In the middle of every difficulty lies opportunity.

—*Albert Einstein*

Yesterday's message discussed those who are troubled by the fact that patients often look better than they feel. However, some people use this to their advantage. I worked with a patient who was able to conceal that he was on HCV treatment, and he went mountain climbing to raise money for charity. Although he didn't feel well, he made it to the summit, which was over 14,000 feet, and he felt good about himself.

Tip for Today: Not everyone will feel like climbing mountains, or even a flight of stairs. Look for opportunities rather than problems. If getting out of bed is hard, then perhaps this is a time to visit with a friend over the phone. If you feel too sick to go to work, use this as a chance to stay at home and watch the birds outside your window. There is always an opportunity somewhere if we just look for it.

Day 91

Look, I really don't want to wax philosophic, but I will say that if you're alive, you've got to flap your arms and legs, you've got to jump around a lot, you've got to make a lot of noise, because life is the very opposite of death.

—*Mel Brooks*

Engaging in physical activity is essential. Moving our bodies helps our muscles, bones, digestive system, heart, brain, attitude, and sleep—just to name a few. Doing anything is better than doing nothing. Make exercise a nonnegotiable element of your commitment to yourself.

> **Tip for Today:** If 30 minutes of daily exercise is too much, can you try 20, 10, or 5 minutes? Park the car at the far end of the parking lot. Take the stairs. Get a walking buddy. Stretch or lift weights when watching your favorite comedy on TV. Flap your arms during every commercial.

WEEK 14

Day 92

Laughter is carbonated holiness.

—Anne Lamott

There is nothing funny about HCV treatment and yet everything about it is funny. After wondering why I could not get my key into the ignition of a car that wasn't even the same make or color as my own, I had a good laugh. Side effects happen and time passes no matter what, and humor makes it easier to deal with the discomfort.

> **Tip for Today:** Surround yourself with people who make you smile. HCV support groups can be laughter jackpots. No one understands better how lousy you feel than a fellow HCV patient who has experienced treatment. Spend a little time in the company of someone who can empathize and before you know it, you won't care that your brain feels like pea soup or that climbing a flight of stairs is like conquering Mt. Everest.

Day 93

Pain is inevitable; suffering is optional.

—Buddhist Proverb

Few things are worse than relentless pain. Coping with pain is part of the human condition, and many have learned how to manage pain and be free from suffering. I knew a patient who endured great pain and hardship during treatment, yet she never suffered. She gathered strength by practicing the Tao, an ancient mind–body spiritual practice.

Tip for Today: Qigong is a technique used in Chinese medicine, purported to restore harmony, energy, and health. Try the following: Standing with your feet shoulder-width apart, toes pointing at a comfortable angle, imagine that you are suspended from a string at the top of your head. Let your hands, arms, and body hang loosely. Breathe naturally. Imagine the energy flowing upward from the earth, through your body, up to the sky, and then back: Sky, body, and earth. Do this for a few breaths.

Day 94

We must learn to reawaken and keep ourselves awake, not by mechanical aids, but by an infinite expectation of the dawn, which does not forsake us in our soundest sleep.

—Henry David Thoreau

This is a lovely quote, but if you are profoundly fatigued, you may need more than the mere expectation of the dawn to keep you awake. Napping may help. Throughout the course of treatment, rule out all medical causes of fatigue such as anemia, low thyroid, depression, diabetes, insomnia, and so on.

Tip for Today: Take short naps—no more than 45 minutes and not close to bedtime. Balance rest with activity. Try to rest before you get too fatigued. Vary activities—don't sit too long or stand too long. Moderate amounts of caffeine in the morning may help you feel more alert and studies have shown improved HCV treatment results among coffee drinkers. A couple of cups of tea or coffee, as long as they don't interfere with your sleep, are safe to use. Unmanageable pain can be exhausting; be sure to seek help for this.

Day 95

Women are like tea bags. You never know how strong they are until you put them in hot water.

—Eleanor Roosevelt

Whether you are a man or a woman, you may be feeling more like pale chamomile than a strong black tea, but the fact that you have made it this far testifies to your strength. Take a moment to reflect on this truth.

> **Tip for Today:** To keep up your strength, be sure you drink plenty of water. For variety, drink tea or mineral water. You can flavor plain water by adding slices of fresh orange, lime, lemon, apple peels, cucumber, or sprigs of mints. Try hot water with lemon, fresh mint, ginger, honey, or herb tea. Experiment with combinations of ingredients.

Day 96

Every morning is like a new reincarnation into this world. Let us take it then for what it is and live each moment anew.

—Paul Brunton

Some HCV patients use medicinal herbs, hoping these will improve their health. In a very large HCV study (HALT-C), conducted by the National Institute of Diabetes and Digestive and Kidney Disease, 23 percent of the participants used herbs at the time of enrollment, with milk thistle being the most commonly chosen. Milk thistle has been used for decades in Germany to reduce inflammation in livers that have been damaged by alcohol or drugs. Encouraged by this, many hope that it will help with other liver diseases, but research has not found any benefit for HCV patients. Unfortunately, all milk thistle is not alike, and the contents of the bottle may not match what is promised on the label. ConsumerLab.com tested 10 milk thistle products, and only one had a sufficient level of active ingredients. In short, you may think you are taking milk thistle, when what you are taking may hardly have any active ingredient. We do not know if milk thistle interacts with telaprevir or boceprevir, but since milk thistle is metabolized by the liver, I'd only take it if medically prescribed.

> **Tip for Today:** If you are interested in milk thistle, talk to your medical provider. Since milk thistle varies between manufacturers, be sure to research before you purchase. Milk thistle is poorly absorbed by the body, so if you take it, choose a formulation and dose that has been tested and certified by a reputable lab. Pharmaceutical-grade supplements are the best. Never use alcohol extracts.

Day 97

The worst thing in the world is to try to sleep and not to.
—*F. Scott Fitzgerald*

Sleep problems are common during HCV treatment. For those who struggle with insomnia, HCV treatment can be especially difficult to endure. Fortunately, there are solutions. Don't assume you have to suffer through sleepless nights; get help and information. Make this a priority.

> **Tip for Today:** Seek professional guidance if you have sleep problems. Never take herbs or sleep medication unless medically prescribed. Some supplements, such as valerian, may be toxic to the liver. If you are considering an herbal blend that claims to improve sleep, make sure valerian is not an ingredient. If you are looking for a natural sleep remedy, try hypnotherapy.

Day 98

A problem is a chance for you to do your best.
—*Duke Ellington*

Rashes are a common HCV treatment side effect, and a side effect that requires great patience. When it comes to aggravation, itching is right up there with insomnia, particularly when itching keeps you awake. Talk to your medical provider if you have skin issues. Redness, swelling, or pus may indicate an infection. The best thing you can do besides getting help is to resist scratching.

> **Tip for Today:** Heat can make skin problems worse. Avoid the sun and extremely hot showers and baths. Keep rooms ventilated and at a temperature of 60°F to 70°F. Wear loose-fitting clothes made from natural, breathable fabrics. Wrap a cold pack in a towel and apply it to itchy areas.

For those on the 28-week plan, congratulations—your treatment is half over. If you made it this far, you can make it the rest of the way, and you are very likely to eradicate HCV permanently. Continue with these readings until your final twelve weeks.

WEEK 15

Day 99

Focus on where you want to go, not on what you fear.
                                                            —Anthony Robbins

During my treatment, I felt deeply anxious nearly every morning while driving to work. I loved my job and could not understand the cause of these feelings. Eventually I was so afraid of the anxiety that it magnified the problem. It took me a month to figure out that these unsettling feelings were a reaction from ribavirin rather than anxiety. Armed with this knowledge, I reminded myself that what I was experiencing was normal and would pass. It helped to practice relaxation exercises while sitting in my car. And although I still felt anxious, I wasn't uneasy about being anxious.

> **Tip for Today:** Learn a few relaxation techniques and practice them regularly. An easy one to try: Sit in a comfortable position. Close your eyes. Notice your breath. Try to bring your breath to your abdomen. Slow down your breathing. When you inhale, say to yourself, *inhaling*, and when you are exhaling say, *exhaling*. Perform this technique for a set period, such as a minute or longer, or for 10 breaths, or until you feel calm entering into your body.

Day 100

Hope is the physician of each misery.
                                                            —Irish Proverb

You have been at this for 100 days. Isn't that incredible! You are made of strong stuff, and you can make it to the end. Just take it easy, be patient, and use all the resources at hand. Never lose hope—it will carry you through.

> **Tip for Today:** Take a moment to look at the past 100 days. What are you doing right? What areas are causing difficulties? Are you utilizing all the resources at hand? Do you need help with anything, either at home, work, or from your medical provider? Identify the biggest problems, and if you can't see solutions, ask for insight, suggestions, and help from others.

Day 101

Always laugh when you can. It is cheap medicine.

—Lord Byron

Not only is laughter cheap medicine, it is readily available, effective and has no side effects. Some patients find it helpful to laugh at themselves—at the silly things they do and say. One patient jokingly put it this way, "It feels like my body has been snatched by aliens, except in this case, the aliens are HCV drugs." Another patient refers to self-injection as "playing darts."

> **Tip for Today:** Find ways to describe your experience. If you can, use humorous descriptions, such as "treatment feels like being at a high altitude, only the view is lousy." Laughing at yourself may help you maintain your perspective and keep you from drifting into darker moods.

Day 102

As you walk and eat and travel, be where you are. Otherwise, you will miss most of your life.

—Buddha

Few of us want to live in the present when we have mouth discomfort. Oral infections may occur during HCV treatment, the most common

> **Tip for Today:** Maintain good oral hygiene. Floss your teeth every day, even if you don't feel like it. Brush your teeth at bedtime and 30 minutes after eating. Include regular trips to the dentist for cleaning and examination as an important part of your HCV treatment regimen. Talk to your medical provider or dentist if you have discomfort or white patches in your mouth or throat. Mild thrush may respond to home remedies such as eating yogurt with live cultures or supplementing with acidophilus. The U.S. National Library of Medicine's PubHealth suggests, "Use a soft toothbrush and rinse your mouth with a diluted 3 percent hydrogen peroxide solution several times a day." Moderate cases require prescription mouthwashes or lozenges. It is best to deal with this early since a rare side effect of the strongest thrush medications is liver damage.

being *thrush*. Thrush, or *candidiasis*, is a fungal infection that is a result of an overgrowth of the mouth's normal flora. Antibiotics and stress may trigger this overgrowth. Signs and symptoms include pain, an odd taste, and white cottage cheese-like lesions anywhere in the mouth.

Day 103

Even as the stone of the fruit must break, that its heart may stand in the sun, so must you know pain.

—*Kahlil Gibran*

You are taking strong medications in order to conquer a fierce virus. Discomfort and pain are sometimes part of the equation. You are doing this so your liver will stay strong so that you will stay alive and see many sunrises. Hold fast to the reasons you are doing this.

Tip for Today: Mild discomfort is common during HCV treatment, but moderate to severe pain requires medical intervention. Also, call your medical provider if you have a fever, nausea, vomiting, or diarrhea. Watch for signs of dehydration, including intense thirst, severe dry mouth, dark urine, dizziness, and pale cold skin. Drink small amounts of whatever you can tolerate, such as water, fruit juice, soda, or sport drinks, and alert your medical provider.

Day 104

A well-developed sense of humor is the pole that adds balance to your steps as you walk the tightrope of life.

—*William A. Ward*

About three months into treatment, one of my patients attended a wedding. He had to stand up to see because his view was blocked by a woman wearing a huge hat. He said, "I was so angry I just wanted to rip the hat off her head." In my nurse role, I sat without judgment, but I could relate. A smile crossed his face as the ridiculousness of his reaction dawned on him. We both laughed.

Tip for Today: Developing a sense of humor includes pursuing pleasure. Using the fingers on one hand, name five things that bring you joy or stir up a memory of pleasure. Perhaps children amuse you, or watching a good football game. Friends, pets, good food, skateboarding as a kid, and thoughts of past or future vacations can inspire pleasant thoughts. Do this frequently. If you can't think of anything that gives you pleasure, talk to your medical provider—it may signal the onset of depression.

Day 105

When the itch is inside the boot, scratching outside of it provides little consolation.

—Chinese Proverb

A frustrating aspect of HCV treatment is that it seems to affect everything we do, even our experiences in the toilet. Some people get hemorrhoids, swollen or inflamed veins in the anal/rectal region. Straining, diarrhea, constipation, and sitting on the toilet for long periods may lead to hemorrhoids. They may itch, hurt, or bleed. Fortunately, there are remedies for these problems.

Tip for Today: If you have hemorrhoids, increase water and fiber intake. Some good fiber sources are wheat bran, prunes, beans, and high-fiber cereals. Talk to your medical provider about over-the-counter laxatives, such as psyllium (Metamucil) and polyethylene glycol 3350 (MiraLax). If you are straining because of hard stools, your medical provider might suggest an over-the-counter stool softener. If hemorrhoids are painful, use specially formulated ointments, and take a pain reliever (unless you have been told otherwise), such as acetaminophen (Tylenol), ibuprofen (Advil, Motrin), naproxen (Naprosyn, Aleve), or aspirin.

WEEK 16

Day 106

Just as the body cannot exist without blood, so the soul needs the matchless and pure strength of faith.

—Mahatma Gandhi

If blood was pouring out of your body, you would get help. What if faith, hope, or determination is hemorrhaging out of your life? These vital aspects of life also need immediate attention. Enduring HCV treatment requires the continual renewal of your physical, emotional, and spiritual health.

> **Tip for Today:** If you are losing faith, hope, or determination, call a friend, spiritual advisor, or therapist. If you are losing blood, the question is how much. Reduced blood-clotting ability is one of the expected side effects of HCV treatment. If you get a cut or nose bleed, it may take longer for the bleeding to stop. If bleeding is excessive or does not stop in 15 minutes, seek medical attention.

Day 107

When angry, count to ten before you speak. If very angry, count to one hundred.

—Thomas Jefferson

When I was on treatment, there were times when I felt cynical, sarcastic, irritable, or resentful. I was not alone in this, as patients related all sorts of stories to me. One wanted to ram another car after the other driver failed to yield at a four-way stop. I slammed my bedroom door when my husband didn't want to go to a movie with me. Although these reactions are common, they are not healthy. We end up feeling awful and pushing others away from us. Road rage is particularly dangerous.

> **Tip for Today:** Don't dismiss your feelings—deal with them. Perhaps counting to 100 is a bit simplistic, but do find a way to keep your emotions from turning into something you may regret later. Try stress reduction techniques. Meditation, physical activity, and support groups can help.

Day 108

If the sky falls, hold up your hands.

—Spanish Proverb

A variation on today's quote is, if the sky falls, hold your neighbor's hand. It is much easier to get through HCV treatment when we are not alone.

> **Tip for Today:** Many of us are happy to help others but would sooner pull out a toenail than ask for help ourselves. However, if no one ever asked for help, we would never experience the good feelings that come from helping another. I think that those who ask for help are the real givers. Try asking for help, and see what happens.

Day 109

Fear less, hope more. Eat less, chew more. Whine less, breathe more. Talk less, say more. Love more, and all good things will be yours.
—*Swedish Proverb*

It would be lovely if we could all follow the advice in today's proverb. A good place to start is to breathe more. Most of the healing and meditation arts in the world emphasize breath work. Focusing on our breath can bring energy, calm, and peace into our lives.

> **Tip for Today:** If you have breathing difficulties, seek immediate medical attention. Shortness of breath is common and may be something you have to put up with during treatment. However, since respiratory problems can be serious, your medical provider needs to determine the scope of the problem. Meditation is a tremendous help for breathing problems aggravated by anxiety.

Day 110

I've learned that even when I have pains, I don't have to be one.
—*Maya Angelou*

On some days, today's quote may seem easier said than done. It is difficult to control our moods during treatment. Our moods affect those around us, which sometimes makes things worse. The trick is to find ways to manage HCV treatment without letting our misery spill over onto others.

Tip for Today: Controlling one's temper is especially important during work. Moodiness and other HCV-related side effects may trickle into the workplace. Legally you do not need to reveal health information. However, if you have not told those you work with that you are on medication that may be altering your performance, it may look like you are developing a work or personality problem. If you prefer not to disclose this information, you may want to explore creative strategies for dealing with your work situation.

Day 111

One cannot think well, love well, sleep well, if one has not dined well.
                                                        —*Virginia Woolf*

Nutrition influences everything we do. If you are tired, make sure you are eating enough, and often enough. Choose high-quality food with lots of nutrients. The human body needs fuel, just as a car needs gas. If you don't eat, you will sputter along until you run out of energy.

Tip for Today: Boost your energy with nutritious food. Protein and complex carbohydrates help to sustain our bodies. Choose foods that are fresh and whole. Try protein shakes with fruit; cottage cheese with sunflower seeds and raisins; almond butter and honey on whole-wheat crackers; sliced turkey on whole wheat bread; humus with tomatoes and cucumbers in a pita; peanut butter on apple slices; cream cheese and celery; a handful of walnuts with your favorite fruit; and low-sodium black beans on a corn tortilla.

Day 112

Be empty of worrying. Why do you stay in prison when the door is so wide open?
                                                        —*Rumi*

Even the most laid back individuals can become champion fretters during HCV treatment. Sometimes we worry about things that aren't worth the anxiety. For instance, abnormal lab results are often normal and expected side effects of HCV drugs. A low white blood cell count does not mean that the immune system is compromised. If you are going to worry, let go of issues that aren't real, present, or helpful to worry about.

> **Tip for Today:** Talk to your medical provider if you are concerned about a lab result or other aspect of your health. It is possible that what you are worrying about is no cause for concern. Make it a policy to get the facts before getting worked up. Freaking out without a good reason is like going to prison before there has even been a trial.
>
> **Note:** For those on a 28-week treatment plan (patients taking boceprevir who meet the criteria of response-guided therapy), skip to Chapter 6, "Readings for the Final 12 Weeks."

WEEK 17

Day 113

A man with outward courage dares to die: A man with inward courage dares to live.

—*Lao Tzu*

Undergoing HCV treatment requires courage. You may lose your stamina, your resolve may be shaky, but despite it all, you are still in the game. If you are tired, in pain, plagued by side effects, hold fast to your courage. It was there the day you administered that first injection; it is here today after the 17th injection; it will be there on the day of the last injection.

> **Tip for Today:** It takes extra courage to make it through treatment if you get headaches. If these are frequent, keep a log to see if there is something causing them. Is there a pattern related to the day of your injection or timing with your pills? Note if you feel especially stressed. Certain foods may trigger headaches, particularly chocolate, coffee, aspartame, aged or fermented foods (aged cheese, vinegars), and foods that have sulfites, monosodium glutamate (MSG), or nitrites (hotdogs, bacon, and lunch meats).

Day 114

Out of discord comes the fairest harmony.

—*Heraclitus*

Life may feel chaotic at times during HCV treatment. All of this will pass. Remain true to your goals of healing. Eventually your life will be restored to harmony.

> **Tip for Today:** Harmony may feel out of reach to anyone with itchy skin. If you are plagued with this, do not scratch. This may lead to worse problems, including infection and increased itchiness. Apply ice or firm pressure to the area. Distract yourself and allow the scratching urge to pass. Moisturize your skin and avoid overly hot showers. Your medical provider may recommend over-the-counter or prescription remedies.

Day 115

We must be willing to give up the life we've planned, so as to have the life that is waiting for us.

—*Joseph Campbell*

Treatment involves giving up a great deal for a relatively short time. After all, what is 24 or 48 weeks compared to a lifetime? Take comfort in the fact that you have travelled a great distance and are getting closer to the life that is waiting for you.

> **Tip for Today:** As you journey toward a healthier life, avoid foraged, wild mushrooms, and raw or undercooked shellfish. These can harbor dangerous toxins that can seriously threaten the liver. Safely handled, fresh raw fish and store-bought mushrooms are fine to eat.

Day 116

A thankful person is thankful under all circumstances. A complaining soul complains even in paradise.

—*Bahá'u'lláh*

It may be hard to muster up thoughts of gratitude during HCV treatment. Although it is precious to think, laugh, and love, these simple pleasures may feel like distant memories. Try thinking about what a privilege it is to be alive and doing HCV treatment.

Tip for Today: Regular bowel movements don't usually make it on to peoples' gratitude lists until they are confronted with constipation. HCV treatment may cause constipation, usually a result of inadequate hydration, immobility, and insufficient fiber in the diet. Constipation is also a side effect of pain medication. Drink plenty of water, particularly warm or hot beverages in the morning. Fruit juices, such as prune, may help. Walk or exercise regularly. Eat a high-fiber diet, including bran, prunes, and raw fruits and vegetables.

Day 117

Live your life as an experiment.

—Chögyam Trungpa Rinpoche

Live your life as an experiment, but use research to guide your health choices. The National Institutes of Health has been interested in the use of herbal remedies among those with liver disease, particularly HCV. Although there has yet to be scientific proof about the benefits of herbs, much more is known about the safety of certain supplements. For instance, black cohosh, comfrey, kava, and vitamin A are particularly toxic to the liver. Milk thistle is generally safe for most people if taken at recommended doses, but research has not shown it to be of any value to those with HCV.

Tip for Today: Apply the same common-sense investigation to dietary supplements as you would to any medicine. Get your facts from experts, not sales people. If you are interested in holistic medicine, consider trying things that don't pass through your liver. Acupuncture, visualization, massage, and affirmations are examples of holistic health that don't require ingesting products.

Day 118

Order is power.

—Henri Frédéric Amiel

Maintaining order will not necessarily bring peace, but living in disorder is like living with mosquitoes buzzing around the ears. Keep the basic structure of your life organized, and everything will be easier. If you always put your car keys or bus pass in the same place, you won't have to look for it anywhere else. If you don't have to spend time looking for something, you'll have extra time for a nap.

Tip for Today: Keep your pills in the same place. If you have to take your pills when you aren't home, use sticky notes or alarms to remind you to take them. When I needed to inject while away from home, I'd put my car keys in an insulated cooler and put the cooler in the fridge. That way I'd remember to take my medication with me. However, I had to leave a note where I normally kept my keys, telling me that the keys were in the cooler; otherwise, I'd think I'd lost them.

Day 119

Just as despair can come to one only from other human beings, hope, too, can be given to one only by other human beings.

—Elie Wiesel

HCV treatment can have moments of despair. Maintaining relationships has tremendous benefits. Do this especially if you feel isolated. If you want to be around people who understand what you are going through, join an HCV group.

Tip for Today: Sexual dysfunction is a particularly cruel side effect of HCV medications because sex is a major part of feeling close to another human being. If you have a sexual partner but don't feel like engaging in sex, find ways to maintain closeness so your partner doesn't feel shut out. Emphasize the fact that this situation is temporary. If you engage in sexual intercourse, remember to use two effective forms of contraception if pregnancy is an issue.

WEEK 18

Day 120

I found that I could find the energy ... that I could find the determination to keep on going. I learned that your mind can amaze your body, if you just keep telling yourself, I can do it ... I can do it ... I can do it!

—Jon Erikson

Sometimes HCV treatment is so tough that we wonder if we'll make it. Fortunately, these moments usually pass for most of us. They pass more quickly if we can find ways to reduce, transcend, or endure discomfort. You know how to do this. The evidence of your strength is the fact that you have made it through another forty days—your third back-to-back journey through this somewhat insane experience.

Tip for Today: Use the three R's to help you through rough spots: review, remind, and recommit. When you review, do some troubleshooting. If you feel like quitting, evaluate what you need in order to keep going. Perhaps more support at home or at work would ease things. Do you need a hepatitis C group? Do you need more help with side effect management? Are your moods getting to you, and if so, perhaps you need medication or a change in medication you are currently taking? Remind yourself of the reasons you are undertaking this journey. Take strides to get what you need to make it to the end, and then recommit to the process.

Day 121

All men whilst they are awake are in one common world: but each of them, when he is asleep, is in a world of his own.

—Plutarch

No one relishes a sleepless night. Add insomnia to a fatigued, grouchy, achy body, and you have a formula for disaster. Fortunately, there are remedies for insomnia, although you may have to try various ones before finding the key to a restful night.

> **Tip for Today:** Try listening to relaxing music or reading something calming before bed. Meditation or a bath may also help. Do not take valerian, an herb touted for insomnia, as there have been reports of liver toxicity.

Day 122

The burden of the self is lightened when I laugh at myself.
—*Rabindranath Tagore*

One of the weird aspects of HCV treatment was how much time I spent thinking about myself. I'd get caught up in rumination. Initially I fretted over the details about HCV treatment, and after a while this pattern became normal. One day I went the entire day without thinking about treatment or how I felt. That day was a gift and after that, I had many moments where I didn't think about what I was going through.

> **Tip for Today:** The side effects of HCV treatment make it hard to ignore how we are feeling. Even small problems such as dry, chapped lips can be a nuisance. Avoid licking your lips, as this will cause them to dry out faster. Keep your lips moist by patting them with a damp soft cloth and then apply lip balm or lubricating jelly. Remove dead cells by rubbing the lips with a soft, dry washcloth or soft toothbrush. Drink lots of water.

Day 123

We don't receive wisdom; we must discover it for ourselves after a journey that no one can take for us or spare us.
—*Marcel Proust*

At this point, HCV treatment may feel less like a journey and more like a trial. You may not realize it, but you are gathering wisdom and strength. Hold fast to those things that guide you safely to the completion of treatment.

> **Tip for Today:** Safety is the number one priority during HCV treatment. Severe or chronic diarrhea is a serious problem that requires medical attention. Mild diarrhea can be relieved with a low-fiber diet. Avoid rich, greasy foods. Dairy products bother some patients, but others state that yogurt improves diarrhea symptoms. Eat easy-to-tolerate foods such as white rice, dry toast, broth-based soups, plain pasta, and crackers. Imodium usually helps with more severe diarrhea.

Day 124

For every minute you are angry you lose sixty seconds of happiness.
—Ralph Waldo Emerson

Anger and agitation are common complaints during HCV treatment. If you feel out of sorts, don't assume that the medicine is causing the problem. For instance, are you sleeping enough? Are you worrying or in pain? Are you constipated? How are your relationships? Is there pleasure in your life? Is laughter part of your health plan?

> **Tip for Today:** If you are irritable, determine the cause; then get help fixing the problem. Rage and violence toward another is never OK. Talk to a professional if you have problems with anger management.

Day 125

Storms make oaks take deeper root. Kites rise highest against the wind—not with it.
—Winston Churchill

Adversity may strengthen us, but the side effects of HCV treatment may weaken our resolve. If you are having problems with memory or concentration, don't give up. Challenge yourself. Stay physically, mentally, and socially active. If you can, avoid passive activities like TV shows that don't stimulate your brain. However, if being a couch potato is the best you can do, then be the best couch potato you can be.

Tip for Today: Challenge your brain. Do arithmetic in your head or on paper rather than use a calculator. Play games or puzzles, such as Sudoku, crossword puzzles, solitaire, and so on. For those with Internet access, type *puzzle, games,* or *brain games* into your search field, and a world of opportunity will open up.

Day 126

No matter what changes take place in the world, or in me, nothing ever seems to disturb the face of spring.

—E. B. White

Life does not stop for medical treatment. Some of the patients I worked with endured incredible hardships in the midst of HCV treatment. Fortunately, good things also occur during treatment. Spring, birthdays, and holidays come every year, no matter what we are doing. Find ways to endure the hard times and enjoy the good ones.

Tip for Today: It is easier to endure HCV treatment with the support of those who have undergone it. If you have access to an HCV group but have yet to attend, this would be a great time to join. If you don't have a group in your area, consider an online group. Keep in mind that not all groups are perfect. Online groups are especially tricky since most are not monitored by medical professionals. However, sometimes patients can support each other in ways that medical professionals cannot.

For those on the 36-week plan, congratulations—your treatment is half over. Continue reading here until your final 12 weeks.

WEEK 19

Day 127

I can tell you that it takes great strength to surrender ... you are going to open to a power that you don't even know, and it is going to come to meet you.

—Marion Woodman

I used to think that surrender was something I had to do at gunpoint. Now I see surrender in a gentler light, such as surrendering a seed to the earth so it can grow. Perhaps there are areas of your life you can surrender, such as some of your workload at home or on the job. Try giving up complex projects; the remaining tasks don't need to be done perfectly.

> **Tip for Today:** If you are feeling tired at work or at home or you are easily overwhelmed, ask those you work or live with to take on some of your regular responsibilities while you are going through treatment.

Day 128

In the world there is nothing more submissive and weak than water. Yet for attacking that which is hard and strong nothing can surpass it.
—Lao Tzu

If you have any doubt about the power of water, think about the Grand Canyon. This amazing wonder was created drop by drop. A single drop of water may not seem like much, but life cannot be sustained without it. Are you drinking enough water?

> **Tip for Today:** If you are having multiple side effects and you are not drinking 9 cups of liquid a day (women) or 13 cups daily (men), try increasing your liquids. You may think you are drinking enough, but when you actually measure it, you may learn that your daily intake of liquids is considerably below the mark. Devise a way to keep track of what you drink. Some patients fill up water bottles every morning with the amount of water they should consume throughout the day.

Day 129

Cancer can take away all of my physical abilities. It cannot touch my mind, it cannot touch my heart, and it cannot touch my soul.
—Jim Valvano

Hepatitis C medication may limit you physically and mentally, but it can't touch your core, that part of you that plunged ahead into treatment. Persistence, patience, and perseverance have kept you going through hard times. Support and good information are effective tools to help manage side effects, and if you aren't using these consistently, now is a good time to start.

> **Tip for Today:** If side effects are causing your patience to wear thin, be sure you are using all the tools available to help you. For instance, mouth sores can be incredibly dispiriting. If you are running out of things to try, consider tea. Black teas, along with some herbal ones are high in tannin. A "used" tea bag placed on a canker sore may provide relief.

Day 130

The man who can drive himself further once the effort gets painful is the man who will win.

—*Roger Bannister*

Some of my patients have accomplished amazing feats during their treatment. One completed a mini-triathlon; another bicycled 200 miles every week. One patient skied all winter, and another never missed his regular gym workout. I walked my dog just about every day, and I thought that was worth an Olympic gold medal. Carrying my own groceries was all I could do the last two weeks of my recent treatment, but I did it.

> **Tip for Today:** Staying fit will help you reach the finish line. However, don't compare yourself to others. Set realistic goals, commit to them, and then make them happen.

Day 131

Originality is unexplored territory. You get there by carrying a canoe— you can't take a taxi.

—*Alan Alda*

Even if you have done HCV treatment before, this is unexplored territory. New situations require new management skills, and new problems require new solutions. The answer to what you need might be somewhere you have never looked before. Keep your eyes open, but do take occasional naps.

Tip for Today: When it comes to side effect management, we may resist dealing with problems because we don't want to add in one more pill. However, there are many ways to manage side effects and other health problems without taking more pills. Acupuncture, acupressure, and other types of bodywork are worth considering if you have the financial means. Some insurance plans pay for these services. If you are fortunate to live in an area that has acupuncture or massage schools, you can look into low-cost clinics.

Day 132

Learn to laugh at your troubles and you will never run out of things to laugh at.

—Lyn Karol

During HCV treatment, a friend was riding his motor scooter on a sunny day. When dusk came, he stopped to remove his sunglasses. Instead, he took out his dentures and then wondered why he was stopped on the side of the road with his teeth out. We got a good laugh over this.

Tip for Today: Laugh at yourself. It's better than the alternatives. If you can't see anything funny about HCV treatment, join a support group. Fellow travelers will show you there is plenty to laugh at.

Day 133

I thank God for my handicaps, for through them I have found myself, my work, and my God.

—Helen Keller

When I don't feel well, I think about others who overcame incredible obstacles. One of my heroes is Dan Caro, who was severely burned when he was a small child. He lost his hands and it took him seven years to learn how to tie his shoes. Although pain is a constant companion, he is now a famous drummer. My temporary conditions seem so minor compared to his and others like him.

> **Tip for Today:** If headaches are handicapping you, talk to your medical provider. Dull, annoying headaches are common, but some patients do get migraines during HCV treatment. Migraine headaches usually need expert advice. No matter what level of headache you may experience, practice stress management and make sure you are well-hydrated. Caffeine may help, cause, or worsen a headache, so if you experiment with this, keep track of how much you use.

WEEK 20

Day 134

Problems arise in that one has to find a balance between what people need from you and what you need for yourself.
—Jessye Norman

The journey through HCV treatment is a time to know what you need to do in order to maintain your health and your resolve. It also is a time to simultaneously push yourself and set limits. This means looking deep inside to find what you are capable of and avoiding doing things that feel burdensome. Only you can know what is good for you.

> **Tip for Today:** Say "no" to those things you don't want to do. You don't have to supply any explanations or apologies. Right now, your health is your main priority. If you are generous with yourself now, you will have more to give in the future.

Day 135

It is part of the cure to wish to be cured.
—Marcus Annaeus Seneca

Perhaps wishing doesn't make it so, but wishing to be cured is an essential part of the healing process. Every time you inject peginterferon or take a pill you are stating your wish to be cured. When you read from this book, attend an HCV group, or see your medical provider, you are committing to your health.

> **Tip for Today:** Maintaining your commitment to health includes eating at regular intervals. Nutritious food is energy. Spread peanut butter on a banana and you have a perfect energy booster. Other healthy snacks are: a handful of almonds and raisins; fruit and yogurt; celery with cream cheese and sunflower seeds; and a flour tortilla with melted mozzarella and sliced tomatoes.

Day 136

There are moments when I feel like giving up or giving in, but I soon rally again and do my duty as I see it: to keep the spark of life inside me ablaze.
—*Etty Hillesum*

Staying positive is one of those things we are implored to try, but if you don't feel positive, it can be torture to try. If you can't muster up any joy, then at least practice acceptance. Even some who have experienced brutal events have found ways to be grateful and joyful. From that perspective, HCV treatment doesn't seem that bad, does it?

> **Tip for Today:** At low points, some patients turn to supplements, hoping these will improve their mood. Resist all temptation to take large doses of vitamins or other supplements. The body is built to use what it needs. At best, your body eliminates the excess, hurting only your budget. At worst, high doses may be toxic to the liver and other organs.

Day 137

Every worthwhile accomplishment, big or little, has its stages of drudgery and triumph: a beginning, a struggle, and a victory.
—*Mahatma Gandhi*

Although successful HCV treatment is helped by patience and a positive attitude, much of treatment seems like sheer drudgery. Going to the doctor, getting lab tests, and managing medication are hardly exciting events. However, they are essential tasks, the value of which is not to be minimized. Each day of HCV treatment is a triumph for your liver and you.

> **Tip for Today:** Victory is more easily felt if you reduce your risk of infections. If you notice bleeding gums, bad breath, or other dental problems, schedule an appointment with your dentist. Some patients get an extra teeth cleaning during treatment. Don't forget to brush and floss.

Day 138

In the stillness of the quiet, if we listen, we can hear the whisper of the heart giving strength to weakness, courage to fear, hope to despair.
                                                                —Howard Thurman

Even if side effects are taking their toll, little gifts of encouragement may grace your path. For instance, the labs measuring your liver enzymes may be normal for the first time in years. Normal alanine aminotransferase (ALT) and aspartate aminotransferase (AST) results suggest that the liver is no longer manufacturing the enzymes that lead to inflammation. Your liver is whispering to you to be strong.

> **Tip for Today:** HCV treatment is hope in a bottle. Treatment is helping your liver, and you can reinforce this by avoiding substances that may damage your liver. Alcohol, high doses of acetaminophen (Tylenol), and certain dietary supplements are some of the substances that can hurt your liver. Abstain from alcohol; don't exceed the recommended doses of medications and supplements, and avoid substances that may be liver-toxic.

Day 139

Apology is a lovely perfume; it can transform the clumsiest moment into a gracious gift.
                                                            —Margaret Lee Runbeck

During my first treatment, I had a few full-fledged temper tantrums in which I behaved very badly. I blamed my family for things that were my fault. Although moodiness and temper flares tend to occur more frequently during HCV treatment, we are still responsible for our words and actions.

> **Tip for Today:** Apology can clear the air for you and everyone around you. Say something such as, "I'm sorry, I am just not my old self." Say it and mean it, even if you don't want to.

Day 140

The big question is whether you are going to be able to say a hearty yes to your adventure.

—Joseph Campbell

If you are losing your enthusiasm for treatment, you are not the first. Suggesting you stay positive is about as reasonable as asking you to smile during dental surgery. However, even if you feel moody and uncomfortable, never forget that you are on a journey toward health. Say a hearty yes or even a feeble one—just keep going unless it isn't wise to do so.

> **Tip for Today:** Depression and anxiety may occur at any point during HCV treatment. Your medical provider should constantly screen for mood changes. If you are already on mood-management medication, the dose may need adjustment or you may need a new or different medication. Talk to your medical provider if the pleasure has gone out of your life.

WEEK 21

Day 141

The period of greatest gain in knowledge and experience is the most difficult period in one's life. Through a difficult period you can learn; you can develop inner strength, determination, and courage to face the problems.

—The 14th Dalai Lama

This may well be one of the most challenging times of your life. You may feel as if you are walking around in a cloud, likely because HCV medications may impair your cognitive function. It feels like brain fatigue, and patients call it *brain fog*. This condition is temporary and will resolve eventually after treatment is finished. Acceptance, determination, and courage will help you manage this frustrating side effect.

> **Tip for Today:** Exercise your brain. The best way to clear the head is with physical activity. Walk, garden, sweep the floor, dance, or try yoga. Don't just sit there—move. Puzzles, reading, learning new things, and games are all fun ways to engage the mind, but exercise is your best bet.

Day 142

Worry does not empty tomorrow of its sorrow; it empties today of its strength.
—Corrie ten Boom

During HCV treatment, worry was my constant companion. Not only did I worry, but I worried that I was worrying. I couldn't seem to stop, so I went into counseling. It helped tremendously because it gave me a place to deposit some of my concerns.

> **Tip for Today:** Get a container and designate it as your worry box. Write down those things that bother you, and put them in the box. Once or twice a day, open the box and allow free worrying, but otherwise, keep the worries in the box. When you find yourself fretting, remind yourself that you put those things in the box. I have a friend who uses a can, and calls it her "God can" (she can't, God can).

Day 142

It is not hard to live through a day, if you can live through a moment. What creates despair is the imagination, which pretends there is a future, and insists on predicting millions of moments, thousands of days, and so drains you that you cannot live the moment at hand.
—Andre Dubus

Sometimes HCV treatment feels as is it will go on forever. There are days when the side effects are especially discouraging; leaving one to wonder if the rest of treatment will be like this. It will get better. Find a way to hold on until it does get better.

> **Tip for Today:** Find ways to relax before you are overly tense. One basic technique is progressive muscle relaxation, which can be done lying down or sitting. Start with your feet: Tense your muscles as tight as you comfortably can. Hold for a few seconds, and then let go. Keep moving up your body, adding muscle groups as you go—feet plus calves; feet, calves, and thighs; feet, calves, thighs, and buttocks. Keep adding muscle groups until you get to your face muscles. After you've let go of every muscle, stay quiet, and breathe, letting go of all tenseness. This is a great exercise to do when trying to go to sleep.

Day 143

Without music, life would be a mistake.

—*Friedrich Nietzsche*

Music has a way of transporting us into another realm. Music can distract us from pain and problems; it can also deepen the connection to our feelings, perhaps intensifying pain, but also providing a place to release what troubles us.

> **Tip for Today:** Spend time listening to some favorite music. If you are feeling tired, try listening to energizing music. If pain is a problem, listen to soothing music. Whatever you are feeling, choose music that reminds you that you are fully alive.

Day 144

Live in the present. Do the things that need to be done. Do all the good you can each day. The future will unfold.

—*Peace Pilgrim*

Patients report a fair amount of self-absorption during treatment. This may be a medication side effect, a consequence of depression and agitation, or a by-product of the isolation that occurs during the process. The best way to combat this is to help others and not isolate yourself. Try to live in the present and take comfort in the fact that the way you are feeling during HCV treatment is temporary.

> **Tip for Today:** Find ways to break the tendency to focus on yourself. Donate money to a favorite nonprofit. Pick up trash on the sidewalk. Call a friend who may be having a hard time. Send a card to a member of the armed services. Hug your kids. Play with your pet. Join a Facebook HCV group and help someone else.

Day 145

If you think you can do a thing or think you can't do a thing, you're right.
—Henry Ford

The mind is a powerful ally. Since we are always thinking, doesn't it make sense to cultivate thoughts of self-confidence rather than indulge negative thoughts of failure? As a friend of mine says, "If you are going to make something up, then make it up rather than down."

> **Tip for Today:** Affirmations are positive statements that offset negative messages. They work even if we don't believe them. We only have to be willing to accept them. Experiment with statements, such as, "I am strong and healthy." "The medication is working." "I am free of pain and worry." Keep affirming even if you don't believe it.

Day 146

A sacred illness is one that educates us and alters us from the inside out, provides experiences and therefore knowledge that we could not possibly achieve in any other way.
—Deena Metzger

Hepatitis C treatment changed me. On good days I was grateful, but on most days I referred to it as an AFOG—Another Freaking Opportunity for Growth (actually, my language was a bit saltier than that). I didn't particularly want to hear that the treatment was an opportunity for growth, but despite myself I did grow from the experience.

> **Tip for Today:** Growth is not something we do alone. If you are feeling lost and overwhelmed or having difficulty coping, talk to a nurse. These professionals have a wealth of information. In addition to the nurse in your medical provider's office, talk to the nurse hotline provided by the pharmaceutical company for the medication you are taking. The pharmacy that supplies your medication may also provide support.

Day 147

Let me tell you the secret that has led me to my goal. My strength lies solely in my tenacity.

—Louis Pasteur

Tenacity and resolve may help you complete treatment, but that doesn't mean you need to white-knuckle it to the end. As you get better at managing side effects, you give yourself the greatest opportunity to ease the process.

> **Tip for Today:** Although this sounds counterintuitive, exercise is one of the most effective ways to combat fatigue. Walking, stretching, or dancing in your kitchen can be very energizing. Be tenacious about your fitness, even if you only move for a minute at a time. Turn on your favorite music and coax your body to move.

WEEK 22

Day 148

Healing is a matter of time, but it is sometimes also a matter of opportunity.

—Hippocrates

Sometimes HCV treatment feels like a nightmare filled with side effects. However, consider this: while your body is having a horrible time, your liver is having a completely different experience. It is getting a break from that ruthless virus and constructing shiny, new liver cells.

> **Tip for Today:** Although your liver is making new cells, your skin is likely having the opposite experience if you are troubled by rashes. If you have itchy skin, don't scratch—advice which is easier said than done. Although scratching may provide temporary relief, it may not stop the source of the itch and could cause an infection. Instead of scratching, use ice. You can confuse the skin's sensory pathways by applying pressure or gently rubbing. Your medical provider may recommend an over-the-counter or prescription remedy. If you scratch yourself while you sleep, wear cotton gloves.

Day 149

There are twelve hours in the day, and above fifty in the night.
—*Marie de Rabutin-Chantal*

Everyone has nights when sleep eludes them, no matter how hard they try. When this happens to you, it's best to find ways to pass the time that are relaxing, keeping your mind off the reality that insomnia has set in. Sleep experts recommend listening to calm music or sounds. I liked listening to audio books as nothing puts me to sleep better than having a story read to me. Avoid watching TV as the light may stimulate the brain into thinking it is morning.

> **Tip for Today:** There are many sources of free or low-cost relaxation recordings. Check the Internet or your local library for audio recordings. If you have a smartphone, iPod, or MP3 player, there are free and low-cost applications specifically designed for relaxation and insomnia. You can download relaxing podcasts to your player. Libraries carry audio books; some even offer pre-loaded MP3 players complete with headphones.

Day 150

Pain is never permanent.
—*Saint Teresa of Avila*

Pain may be temporary, but the pain of mouth sores can feel like an eternity. Although many people never have a single mouth sore during their entire HCV treatment, others develop them early and often. When I had mouth sores, I worked closely with my medical provider to learn ways to prevent the sores or manage them once they occurred. If you are plagued by mouth problems, talk to your medical provider.

Tip for Today: A variety of mouth sore solutions are available by prescription. Often called *Magic Mouthwash*, the ingredients vary between prescribers. An over-the-counter version uses a teaspoonful of an antacid such as milk of magnesia (magnesium hydroxide) or Mylanta (aluminum and magnesium hydroxides) with a teaspoonful of liquid Benadryl (diphenhydramine). Swish, then spit or swallow four to six times daily. If mouth sores are severe, ask your medical provider about prescription-strength liquid numbing agent that uses viscous lidocaine.

Day 151

To forgive is to set a prisoner free and discover that the prisoner was you.
—Lewis B. Smedes

I had to do a fair amount of apologizing during my HCV treatment. However, I also had to learn to overlook others' mistakes. People had no idea how lousy I felt. That wasn't their fault. I had to give up my expectations that others would understand how hard HCV treatment was, and forgive them when my feelings got hurt.

Tip for Today: Forgiveness is a powerful tool and can keep you safe. For instance, if you get annoyed easily when driving, formulate a policy that will help you keep your anger in check. Try this: forgive five people for their driving errors, and don't get upset until the sixth infraction. Or, decide you will not get mad at the way anyone drives until you are home and not behind the wheel. Another suggestion: imagine that the person behind the wheel just found out that they lost their job or heard other bad news. Then visualize their safe passage.

Day 152

A sense of humor is the ability to understand a joke—and that the joke is oneself.

—*Clifton Paul Fadiman*

The inability to concentrate is a frustrating HCV treatment side effect and there is not always a good way to manage it. Humor makes it bearable. I told myself that I had acute interferon-induced attention-deficit disorder. It's not an official medical disorder, but anyone who has been through it knows it is real.

Tip for Today: Talk to your medical provider if you have problems concentrating. Various medications may help. Be sure you are getting sufficient sleep and exercise. Being organized and keeping lists is helpful. Above all, laugh at yourself.

Day 153

Everybody needs a hug. It changes your metabolism.

—*Leo Buscaglia*

Isolation is a huge problem during HCV treatment. Humans need to be connected to each other, and too much time away from others can force us into a world where all we listen to is our own misery. Human contact, whether in the form of a hug, a conversation, a smile, or a shared experience, can transform desolation into consolation.

Tip for Today: Massage has miraculous healing properties. It helps us feel connected and is a fantastic stress-buster. It's great for muscle pain and other body aches. If you can't afford a professional massage, see if there is someone in your area that is learning this art and needs volunteers. Look for coupons on the Internet or in the paper; ask for a discount. Some massage therapists will barter if you have a service that you can exchange.

Day 154

Thousands have lived without love, not one without water.
—W. H. Auden

Love is vital, but useless if you don't have enough water. Good hydration will help with HCV treatment side effects, such as fatigue, dizziness, and dry skin. Strive to drink the amount of water recommended for you.

> **Tip for Today:** Cornell researchers discovered that if beverages are served in short, wide glasses, people drink about 30 percent more. People drink less when beverages are served in tall, skinny glasses. What kind of glass are you using?

WEEK 23

Day 155

The aim of the wise is not to secure pleasure, but to avoid pain.
—Aristotle

So often, we are told that gain requires pain or that pain is the threshold to opportunity. Although there is wisdom in these maxims, when it comes to physical pain, this is simply not true. Pain may build character, but it is a signal that something is wrong. There are many ways to treat pain, and if you are experiencing pain, tell your medical provider. You do not have to suffer.

> **Tip for Today:** Your nurse or doctor may ask you to rate your pain on a scale of 0 to 10. You may wonder, "If I say 4, maybe I won't get help for the pain." The goal is to have you at zero or one. Be honest about your needs. If the doctor prescribes something that is not effective, then it is time to try something else. Note: if you are prescribed a drug in which acetaminophen is an ingredient, such as Vicodin or Norco, be sure you calculate the total amount you are taking, including all over-the-counter and prescription drugs. Ask your medical provider how much acetaminophen you can take safely. Most liver experts recommend 650 mg every four hours or 1000 mg every six hours for their adult patients.

Day 156

The days of our lives, for all of us, are numbered. We know that. And yes, there are certainly times when we aren't able to muster as much strength and patience as we would like. It's called being human.
—Elizabeth Edwards

The expression, "our days are numbered" is not a consoling one. However, take comfort in the fact that the days of your HCV treatment are numbered. This will not go on forever. The fact that you have endured 156 days already proves how strong you are. You may be feeling weak, but since you lasted this long, it shows you are resilient.

Tip for Today: If like me, you started this treatment with the full intention of conquering all side effects, then by now you may have learned just how human you are. On one hand, hepatitis C treatment is a monumental challenge; on the other, it is a constant reminder that you are human. Be gentle with yourself during the difficult times. The more forgiving you are of yourself and others, the easier this journey will be.

Day 157

The only way around is through.

—Robert Frost

It's been said that if you are going through hell, keep walking. Eventually you will come out the other side. The same can be said about HCV treatment—the way out is by going through it. Take comfort in the fact that you have proven yourself to be hardy enough to make it through.

Tip for Today: Apologies to Robert Frost, but today's quote brings to mind constipation, particularly since this condition can make one feel sluggish. Assuming you have sufficient water, fiber, and exercise in your daily routine, then it may be time to consider over-the-counter assistance. Start with something gentle such as polyethylene glycol 3350 (MiraLax), psyllium (Metamucil), partially hydrolyzed guar gum (Benefiber), or methylcellulose (Citrucel). If you still have a problem, ask your medical provider or pharmacist to recommend an effective over-the-counter laxative. If you have nausea, vomiting, or stomach pain, consult with your medical provider before taking a laxative.

Day 158

It is his restraint that is honorable to a person, not their liberty.
—John Ruskin

HCV treatment affects some people's ability to deal with anger. Carrying resentments is like trying to live with a ball and chain; it feels awful. Even worse is when we lash out at another. If you are bothered by resentments, talk to a trusted friend, therapist, clergy person, or medical provider. If depression or anxiety are frequent, unwanted companions, medication may help if these problems are treatment-induced.

Tip for Today: If you feel strongly about something and are tempted to write a letter to the newspaper or to a friend or family member, think twice about it. Restraint of pen and tongue can keep us out of trouble. E-mails, letters, and confrontations are best done when feeling rational and detached. If these issues are truly important, they will still be there when you are done with treatment.

Day 159

There are two ways to live your life—one is as though nothing is a miracle, the other is as though everything is a miracle.
—Albert Einstein

Miracles are all around us. Medicine is a miracle. So is hope. It is a miracle that you willingly take medication into your body, investing nothing less than your entire life into HCV treatment. In short, you are a miracle.

Tip for Today: Spend some time thinking about the miracles in your life. Write them down in case you forget them. If you can't identify any miracles, call some friends and ask them to name some miracles.

Day 160

The soul that has no established aim loses itself.
                    —*Michel Eyquem de Montaigne*

This is your fourth back-to-back forty-day trip into this strange and wild experience. If you have any lingering doubts about your ability to endure difficulty, now is a good time to let these go. You have proven that you are resilient.

> **Tip for Today:** The reason why it is important to review our goals as we go along is that it is easy to get distracted from them. This is particularly true if you are having a hard time with side effects. In preparation for the next 40 days, review your goals, remind yourself of the reasons why you are undertaking this journey, and recommit to the process.

Day 161

Endurance is one of the most difficult disciplines, but it is to the one who endures that the final victory comes.
                                        —*Buddha*

Endurance gets shakier under intense pain, particularly for migraine sufferers. Although some patients are afflicted with migraines during HCV treatment, many experience less severe but relentless headaches. They are often described as dull, near-constant, unwanted companions. More than a few patients have described this side effect as a headache that isn't quite a headache. To me it felt like a tropical storm that never became a hurricane.

> **Tip for Today:** If you have a dull headache, consider alternative medicine, such as acupressure. Try pinching the deep tissue at the crook of the "V" between your thumb and forefinger. Hold for at least seven seconds. Repeat on the other hand and do as often as necessary.

WEEK 24

Day 162

For all that has been, thanks; to all that will be, yes.
—Dag Hammarskjöld

Assuming the length of your treatment is 48 weeks, you have completed half of your injections. The fact that you have come this far proves that you have what it takes to make it for 24 weeks—which is all you need to do to get to the finish line.

For those of you on a 24-week plan, this is your last peginterferon injection. You may get more out of this book if you skip ahead to the last week's readings. You still have a week of pills to take, so you aren't quite done, but go ahead and celebrate the milestone of no more injections.

Tip for Today: No matter where you are in the course of treatment, take a moment to give thanks and to recommit to what is ahead. Be sure you are up to date on all laboratory tests. If you don't have any tests scheduled for this time point, call your medical provider and ask when these will be ordered.

Day 163

The block of granite, which was an obstacle in the path of the weak, becomes a stepping-stone in the path of the strong.
—Thomas Carlyle

Are there any obstacles on your path? This is a good time to look at the side effects that hinder you the most. What are your biggest problems? Fatigue, depression, anxiety, insomnia, poor attitude, pain, relationships, work, loss of enthusiasm, inability to concentrate, and low libido are some of the biggest concerns. It may feel overwhelming at times, but take heart—most of the side effects of HCV treatment can be managed. Even if these side effects have not been adequately managed, don't lose hope.

Tip for Today: Problems have solutions. List your major problems and ask for suggestions on how to manage these. Pick the problem that bothers you the most and get help for it. If medical issues are on your list, discuss these with your medical provider.

Day 164

Two men look out the same prison bars; one sees mud and the other stars.
—Frederick Langbridge

It always amazes me when patients manage to put a positive spin on a side effect. A few of my patients actually liked the hair loss that accompanied HCV medications—one because her hair was very thick, another because she wanted to experiment with a short haircut.

Tip for Today: If your hair is dry or brittle, don't wash it as often as you normally do. Reduce the heat settings on dryers or electric curlers. Even better, stop using hair dryers or switch to one made from tourmaline ($20–$30).

Day 165

When I find myself fading, I close my eyes and realize my friends are my energy.
—Unknown

HCV treatment can be a lonely experience. People around you have no idea of what you are experiencing unless they have been through it themselves. However, just because they don't completely understand doesn't mean that they can't care about you deeply and help you to walk through rough times.

Tip for Today: Ask a friend or family member to go for a walk. Pick a nice flat place to stroll, perhaps with a place to sit down if you get tired. It doesn't need to be a long walk. A little exercise and companionship can have all sorts of benefits. Consider setting a date to do this regularly.

Day 166

You've got to jump off cliffs all the time and build your wings on the way down.

—Ray Bradbury

HCV treatment is like jumping off a cliff, sometimes every day, or even every hour. The fact that you made it this far is evidence that you are flapping your wings.

> **Tip for Today:** Jumping off cliffs is one thing, but dry mouth and bad breath are nuisances. Chew on crisp foods, such as apples, jicama, carrots, or cucumber. The saliva production combined with the scouring action of the crisp produce is good for your teeth.

Day 167

No one is as capable of gratitude as one who has emerged from the kingdom of night.

—Elie Wiesel

Gratitude is more than a concept—it is a choice. When we are thankful, we say "yes" to the gift of life. It does not negate our pain—it softens it, making it easier to bear.

> **Tip for Today:** Gratitude in daylight is easy compared to how we feel during the loneliness of the night. If you have trouble sleeping, do an alphabet gratitude list. For each letter of the alphabet, beginning with A, name something for which you are grateful. If you are still awake when you get to the letter X, you may be stumped. Feel free to use my gratitude item—"xtra" health because of a life without hepatitis C.

Day 168

The lowest ebb is the turn in the tide.

—Henry Wadsworth Longfellow

Today is a day to celebrate—you are half-way through. Take a moment to acknowledge your amazing accomplishment. If you are wondering if treatment will get harder, it doesn't usually. There may be ups and downs but you have already proved that you are capable of meeting these challenges.

> **Tip for Today:** Plan a celebration. Go all out—maybe even put three maraschino cherries in your tonic water. You don't need to spend a lot of time or money rejoicing; just be sure to mark the occasion, for even if you feel low, know that the tide has turned.

For those on a 36-week treatment plan (patients taking boceprevir who meet the criteria of response-guided therapy), skip to Chapter 6, "Readings for the Final 12 Weeks."

5

●●●●●●○

Readings for Weeks 25 through 36

Day 169

Humor is the instinct for taking pain playfully.

—*Max Eastman*

Here is an uplifting fact: you have more treatment behind you than ahead of you. At this point, you may find that treatment gets tedious. Don't let side effects or boredom derail you from reaching your goal. Maintain your resolve and your humor.

Tip for Today: Maintaining resolve may be easier said than done, particularly if you are feeling miserable. Find ways to put a humorous spin on your experience. For instance, on injection days, say, "Today I get to practice being a pin cushion, which will come in handy if a tailor is looking for help" or, "My skin is so raw I might be able to pick up extra money as a model for Dermatology Illustrated." Positive affirmations, such as "I welcome the benefits of peginterferon" are essential tools, but humor is more fun. Use both.

Day 170

We either make ourselves miserable or we make ourselves strong. The amount of work is the same.

—Carlos Castaneda

Loss of appetite during HCV treatment is common, which may cause weight loss. Since many of us have a few extra pounds, this isn't always a bad thing. However, losing weight and losing your appetite are two different issues. First, food is fuel, so we need to eat enough calories for the body to function. Second, rapid weight loss can rob the body of muscle mass rather than just fat loss. You may feel miserable, but you need to stay strong. If weight or appetite loss is problematic, discuss this with your medical provider.

Tip for Today: If you are struggling with food or weight issues, try eating small portions at frequent intervals. Every couple of hours, snack on combinations of foods that are high in protein and calories. Some suggestions: Crackers with a slice of cheese, an apple with peanut butter, celery or bagel with cream cheese, cottage cheese and sunflower seeds, pita bread and hummus, tortilla with melted cheese, a pear with almond butter, tortilla chips with bean dip, a fruit smoothie or milk shake with protein powder, fruit and full-fat yogurt.

Day 171

The feeling of sleepiness when you are not in bed, and can't get there, is the meanest feeling in the world.

—Edgar Watson Howe

Sometimes fatigue is so intense that you may consider giving up just about anything for a place to lie down. My car was my favorite nap place. I'd lock the doors, put the driver's seat back as far as it would go and shade my eyes from the sun. It was uncomfortable, but the fatigue was so awful that it was worth the discomfort.

Tip for Today: A 20 to 30 minute nap can work wonders; even a minute or two may help. If you are concerned about sleeping too long, set the alarm on your cell phone or watch.

Day 172

Always fall in with what you're asked to accept. Take what is given, and make it over your way. My aim in life has always been to hold my own with whatever's going. Not against: with.

—*Robert Frost*

Brain fog is incredibly frustrating because it interferes with nearly everything. The real nuisance is that once you are already cognitively impaired you can't access your brain to help you out of the fog. Although it is a nuisance, fighting against it makes it worse. Acceptance clears the way for the emergence of practical solutions when your brain isn't operating like it used to. Getting annoyed blocks the way out of the fog.

Tip for Today: One way to manage brain fog is by developing reliable habits and sticking to them. Prevent a pile-up of paper. If you pay your bills as soon as you get them, they won't get lost or forgotten. You can automate the process by using secure online payments. Many feel it is safer than mailing a check. You save the price of the stamp and avoid costly late fees.

Day 173

It's important I surround myself with people who make me happy.

—*Adam Sandler*

Few things feel better than being surrounded by people who love us and make us happy. Scientific studies have shown that happiness improves the immune system. A positive social network is a safe, inexpensive way to boost your immune function.

Tip for Today: Experience tells us that being around people who make us unhappy is a huge energy drain. If there are people in your life that are especially difficult to be with, consider limiting your exposure to them. If you live or work with them, find ways to take care of yourself such as by detaching emotionally.

Day 174

Sex at age ninety is like trying to shoot pool with a rope.

—George Burns

This George Burns quote sums up what patients may experience during HCV treatment. The sexual problems that patients encounter vary, ranging from lack of interest to pain during intercourse. Some men complain of erectile dysfunction; some women complain of vaginal dryness. The ones who aren't complaining are too sick or tired to complain.

Tip for Today: If sex was an important aspect of your relationship with your partner, then sexual problems may be a huge issue during HCV treatment. Be sure to discuss this with your partner. You may not want to talk about it, but it is important that you make room for your partner to bring it up. Good communication is important to the health of relationships.

Day 175

Choose rather to be strong of soul than strong of body.

—Pythagoras

Treatment doesn't mean we completely surrender to feeling weak, either in body or soul. Staying physically strong is difficult but straightforward. Losing spiritual strength may be more problematic since for many, a strong spirit is the foundation of physical and mental health.

Tip for Today: Spend a quiet moment asking this question: What does my spirit need? If no answer appears, try writing in a journal, walking in nature, or talking with a wise friend. Ask the question before you fall asleep and see if an answer comes to you in a dream. Once you know what you need, take action. Develop a regular practice; spiritual health needs regular exercise.

WEEK 26

Day 176

Peace is only a thought away, and all we have to do to access it is to silence the voice of our dominating left mind.

—*Jill Bolte Taylor*

Today's quote comes from a brain scientist who experienced a massive stroke when she was 37 years old. In *My Stroke of Insight*, Taylor describes how the experience leads her to discover a great deal about herself and how her brain works. Some HCV patients find that treatment teaches them much and is an opportunity to develop new coping skills.

Tip for Today: Listen to what you are saying to yourself. Are you engaging in negative self-talk? If you are having difficulty letting go of negative thoughts or feelings, try replacing them with positive ones. For example, if you tell yourself you can't make it through another day, try saying, "I made it through another day and I will make it through the next one." If you are feeling tired, try saying, "I am getting my energy back."

Day 177

Nothing cures insomnia like the realization that it's time to get up.

—*Author Unknown*

After a night of tossing and turning, a cruel reality sets in—sleep comes when it is time to get up. It never fails to amaze me that I can function the next day on very little sleep, albeit poorly. A nap and some caffeine may be necessary in order to do this. Fortunately, the latest research shows that caffeine may be beneficial for the liver, although using it late in the day can interfere with sleep. If you are tired, be careful when driving.

Tip for Today: The scent of lavender may promote sleep. Assuming you aren't allergic to it, try spraying lavender on your pillow case and sheets. Apply lavender oil to your wrists or temples. Place a lavender sachet inside your pillow. Although the benefits of lavender have not been well researched, it is not harmful and it smells wonderful.

Day 178

She would rather light candles than curse the darkness and her glow has warmed the world.

—Adlai Stevenson

Some days can feel very dark during treatment. Rather than curse the darkness, find ways to brighten your mood. You can always ask a friend to light some candles for you. Or, you can turn your thoughts to others by lighting a candle for someone who is struggling.

Tip for Today: Qigong can brighten a dark mood. Here is a variation of the practice suggested on Day 93 that can help if you are too fatigued to stand: Sit in a comfortable, straight-back chair with your feet flat on the ground. Relax your hands, palms facing upward, resting on your lap. Imagine that you are suspended from a string at the top of your head. Breathe naturally. Picture the energy flowing upward from the earth, through your body, up to the sky, and then back through your open hands, through your body and back to earth. Do this for a few breaths.

Day 179

We count our miseries carefully, and accept our blessings without much thought.

—Chinese Proverb

I worked with a patient whose husband died unexpectedly while she was going through treatment. He was her sole support. She also lost her house and medical insurance because of his death. She had cirrhosis and was quite sick even before treatment. She did not quit until her doctor told her that she wasn't responding to HCV therapy and that she had to stop.

Although this patient was heroic, she was terrified before starting treatment. She was so fearful that I didn't think she was going to try it, but she prevailed over her fear. She was an inspiration—through treatment and pain. She said to me, "Once you have lost everything, life is easier to live. You know you can survive anything."

Tip for Today: Much of what you have lost during treatment is temporary. Count your blessings, not your miseries.

Day 180

In terrible moments, in moments of revolution, of war or repression, of illness or death, people react with incredible strength.

—Isabel Allende

Even without knowing you, I know how strong you are. If there is any doubt in your mind about how resilient you are, think about this: You have been taking HCV medications for nearly half a year. That's a long time, and yet, here you are, still in the race. This speaks volumes about your strength.

Tip for Today: Keep fortifying your strength. Physical activity helps with a variety of side effects and is the best defense against fatigue. Be sure to move and stretch throughout the day.

Day 181

Life isn't about waiting for the storm to pass. It's about learning to dance in the rain.

—Usually attributed to Vivian Greene

Some days, HCV treatment feels like a thunderstorm; other days like a gentle rain. Some side effects are huge and some are small. It is often the accumulation of the little side effects that weighs heavily.

> **Tip for Today:** Dry, brittle fingernails are hardly a crisis, but you don't have to grin and bear it, especially since there are things you can do that may help. Limit the amount of time your hands are immersed in water, particularly hot water. Wear gloves when washing the dishes, preparing food, and gardening. Apply hand creams frequently, especially after you wash your hands. Apply nail strengtheners to nails. Stay well-hydrated by drinking lots of water. At bedtime, saturate your hands with A & D ointment, a heavy cream, coconut oil, or shea butter; sleep with cotton gloves.

Day 182

The call of the moon and forest was irresistible. The storms of the monsoon season also called to me ... When I hear it now, I pause ... and I listen with awe and passion.

—Thich Nhat Hanh

Nature can heal us with its sheer beauty, even in the dead of winter. Are you cooped up all day? Have you taken a moment to go outside, look around you, and breathe in the fresh air? Even if you live in a big city, you can find a corner of natural wonder to admire.

> **Tip for Today:** Go to a park, community garden, or other outdoor site, and spend time absorbing the marvels. If the weather is bad, briefly open a window or relish nature from a sheltered location. Watch a nature program on TV; check out the DVD series *Planet Earth* for some especially incredible views of the world. You can rent these or borrow them from your library.

WEEK 27

Day 183

A human being is only breath and shadow.

—Sophocles

Borrowing from Sophocles' quote, one could say that HCV treatment is largely breath and shadow. Some days it may feel as if you are walking in darkness, and the only light is the assurance that treatment will not go on forever. However, as long as you are breathing, there is life. So, if the going gets tough, ask yourself, "Am I breathing?" As long as the answer is yes, there is hope.

> **Tip for Today:** Serious breathing problems rarely occur during HCV treatment, but call 911 if you can't breathe. The most common treatment-related respiratory problems are congestion or shortness of breath with exertion. Tell your medical provider if you have any breathing problems; your provider may order some diagnostic tests or prescribe medication for this.

Day 184

Doubt is uncomfortable, certainty is ridiculous.

—Voltaire

While taking HCV medications, I had moments when my family told me I was acting strangely. I reacted defensively, steadfast in my belief that I was the only one with a hold on reality. In retrospect, I can see that this hold was fragile, but I clung to it, unaware that my clinging was making matters worse.

> **Tip for Today:** Try not to get stuck in your head, wondering if you are losing your mind or if others have gone bonkers. Create some space for yourself—to breathe, console, and heal from the chaotic thoughts that often are part of HCV treatment.

Day 185

My friends are my estate.

—Emily Dickinson

HCV treatment can be a lonely experience. Sometimes we feel that others don't understand us. We may not be aware of our moods, unconsciously pushing others away from us. We need support more than ever; yet, it is too easy to let it slip away. We need our friends at a time when we may be acting the most unfriendly.

Tip for Today: Are you feeling isolated? Spend time with friends or family doing activities that bring you pleasure. If going out seems like too much effort, ask them to bring over your favorite food and have a meal together in your home. Whatever you do, don't tire yourself out by cleaning the house first. A good friend doesn't care if there are dirty dishes in the sink, and a great friend might offer to wash them. The best friends are there even when you are grouchy.

Day 186

My life has been filled with terrible misfortunes—most of which never happened.

—Mark Twain

The first time I went through HCV treatment, I looked for help on the Internet. I joined a few online hepatitis C groups, hoping to pick up tips to make my treatment easier. I quickly learned that although there was support and wisdom, there was also complaining and misinformation. I took everything with a grain of salt, and in time, I learned what sites and people to trust.

Tip for Today: If you want more information and support, look at some of the websites listed in the Resources guide at the end of this book. For reliable information, my favorite website is www.hcvadvocate .org. If you want to join a discussion group and are new to web-based groups, spend time reading posts and getting to know people before jumping in. Facebook, Google, and Yahoo all have many hepatitis C groups from which to choose. Sample one and if a group doesn't meet your needs, then try another one.

Day 187

It is part of the human spirit to endure and give a miracle a chance to happen.

—Jerome Groopman, MD

The miracle happened the day you began HCV treatment. It is likely that you have endured quite a bit by now, extending the miracle as you continue to take the medications. Although there are no guarantees, the fact that you have made it this far demonstrates your ability to make it through the rest of treatment.

Tip for Today: The trick to treatment is to make it safely through to the end. The ingredients for success include good side effect management, support, and sheer tenacity. However, some days these may not be enough. Remind yourself, or ask others to remind you, of this simple truth: You made it this far and you can make it the rest of the way. The human spirit is amazing, and it will carry you through the rest of treatment.

Day 188

When it is dark enough you can see the stars.

—*Ralph Waldo Emerson*

After this many months of treatment, life may feel dark and heavy because of the relentless effects of HCV medications. However, there is no other proven way to get rid of HCV. The odds are in your favor that you will beat this virus. In the meantime, when life seems dark, look for the stars.

Tip for Today: Although today's reading suggests focusing on the delights that can be seen in the dark, it is a good reminder to pay attention to any visions problems you may be having. Although these problems are uncommon, if you notice any changes in your eyesight, such as blurry or loss of vision, notify your medical provider immediately. Most vision problems are minor and easily addressed, but these are symptoms you do not want to ignore.

Day 189

It is by going down into the abyss that we recover the treasures of life. Where you stumble, there lies your treasure.

—*Joseph Campbell*

Something that is rarely discussed is that some incredible moments may occur during HCV treatment. We are so vulnerable that joy breaks through our wounds at the most unexpected moments. These are moments of grace.

> **Tip for Today:** You are more likely to experience the gifts that life bestows if you look for them, rather than wait for the gifts to come to you. Try to stay in the present. Don't fight treatment. Wear it like a loose garment rather than a straightjacket.

WEEK 28

Day 190

When we need these healing times, there is nothing better than a good long walk. It is amazing how the rhythmic movements of the feet and legs are so intimately attached to cobweb cleaners in the brain.
—Anne Wilson Schaef

I walked nearly every day during my HCV treatment. Sometimes my pace was so slow that my dog was practically pulling me on the leash. That didn't matter; all that mattered was that I was still moving. Motion meant that I was alive.

> **Tip for Today:** This week pick a place to walk that is surrounded by beauty, such as a park, trail, or favorite street. Take your time; it's not a race. Even if you only walk for 10 minutes, you can sit for another 10 minutes and absorb the wonder of the world.

Day 191

The art of life is the art of avoiding pain; and he is the best pilot, who steers clearest of the rocks and shoals with which it is beset.
—Thomas Jefferson

I worked with quite a few patients who were in pain. Some believed that they had to tough it out, so they refused pain medication. Some just didn't want to take any more pills, an understandable choice, but one that kept them in pain. Patients who are in recovery for addiction are appropriately concerned about taking pain relievers. However, pain stresses the body and takes all the pleasure out of living. Appropriate pain management can restore hope and joy.

Tip for Today: If you are in pain, tell your medical provider. Be open and honest about your concerns. Mention previous experiences with pain management, whether positive or negative. If you don't like how you feel on pain medications, discuss strategies that will reduce side effect risks, such as taking a low dose with gradual increases. Another strategy is to get the pain under control and then decrease the dosage. Pain control offers many choices, particularly if addiction is an issue. Nondrug pain management techniques, such as acupuncture, visualization, massage, and meditation may offer additional relief.

Day 192

However long the moon disappears, some day it must shine again.
—Nigerian Proverb

Sometimes, after a spell of bad weather, we may wonder if the sun will ever shine again. Likewise, during HCV treatment, it may seem hard to believe that you will ever feel good again. Believe me, one day you will get your body and your life back. If you eliminate HCV, you may come out ahead.

Tip for Today: Little things can bring pleasure. Step outside and look at the moon. Spend Sunday afternoon watching a football game. Relax in a comfortable chair and listen to your favorite music. Don't worry about getting anything accomplished— treatment is your work.

Day 193

The ultimate measure of a man is not where he stands in moments of comfort and convenience, but where he stands at times of challenge and controversy.
—Martin Luther King, Jr.

We already know how you measure up—you are mighty. Look at how you have stuck with treatment and how much you have endured because of it. Have you stopped to think how strong and determined you are?

Tip for Today: An irony of treatment is that minor side effects can cause the biggest challenges. For instance, dry lips may be turning into a painful annoyance. If this hasn't been responding to previous suggestions, try increasing your exfoliation and moisturizing routine. Rub your lips gently with a soft, dry washcloth or fine facial exfoliating mud. Apply heavy lip balm or ointment, such as Aquaphor Lip Repair, ChapStick Overnight Lip Treatment, or Nivea's A Kiss of Moisture. Reapply lip treatment throughout the day.

Day 194

When I hear somebody sigh, "Life is hard," I am always tempted to ask, "Compared to what?"

—*Sydney J. Harris*

Sometimes life seems hard because of our circumstances; other times it is hard because of our perspective. If you are having a difficult time, take a moment to figure out if it is because of your attitude or your situation. Regardless of the cause, the solution is the same—adjust your attitude.

Tip for Today: If your attitude is defying adjustment, try stress-relieving techniques used in Chinese medicine. This ancient art applies pressure to trigger points, helping to unblock and restore the energy flow. The following technique is purported to stimulate endorphins, cortisol, and adrenaline: Using your thumb and index finger, lightly squeeze your earlobes. Massage your lobes, gently moving along the ear's outer rim.

Day 195

Pure water is the world's first and foremost medicine.

—*Slovakian Proverb*

Patients state that when they don't get enough fluids, their side effects are more noticeable. Dehydration can cause or worsen fatigue. Stay hydrated, even if you don't feel like drinking liquids. Some people don't like to drink water; some get bored with it, and if you aren't sufficiently hydrated, find ways to increase your water intake.

> **Tip for Today:** Plain water isn't the only way to stay hydrated. Although juice and soda are not the best choices, they are better than not drinking. You can dilute juice by adding carbonated water. During my treatment, I craved tonic water with a maraschino cherry. On evenings out, I'd go all out and have two of these.

Day 196

But only the dance is sure! Make it your own.
                        —*William Carlos Williams, "The Dance"*

Hundreds of thousands of patients have gone through HCV treatment, but no one will have the same experience as you. This is your dance—and you can do this any way you desire—just don't stop dancing.

> **Tip for the Day:** You may not feel like doing much, but keeping active is essential. Your bones, joints, muscles, brain, and mental health need a certain amount of regular physical activity in order to function at their best. You may not feel like doing much, but do it anyway. A slow walk around the block is better than doing nothing.

WEEK 29

Day 197

Anything in life that we don't accept will simply make trouble for us until we make peace with it.
                        —*Shakti Gawain*

Life is especially hard when we can't seem to break free from something that is troubling. Resentments, worry, pain, relationships, fear, and sadness can burden us so much that we may wonder how we can make it through the day, let alone to the end of HCV treatment. However, there are ways to lighten the load, such as by talking to friends, professionals, and others who have been through treatment or other challenges.

Tip for Today: If something is bothering you, try the following prayer:

God, grant me the serenity to accept the things I cannot change, courage to change the things I can, and wisdom to know the difference.

—*The Serenity Prayer*, Attributed to Reinhold Niebuhr

Day 198

Healing may not be so much about getting better, as about letting go of everything that isn't you—all of the expectations, all of the beliefs—and becoming who you are.

—*Rachel Naomi Remen*

Healing from hepatitis C can be a violent process, or a merely annoying one. However, sometimes the nuisances are hard to deal with, because they don't demand our immediate attention. Healing includes learning to live with the unpleasant but minor side effects that accompany HCV treatment. Healing also involves learning the difference between a truly minor problem and a minor problem that is a symptom of a more serious one.

Tip for Today: Some patients experience an unpleasant taste in their mouth, often described as a metallic flavor. This common annoyance is usually not cause for alarm but could indicate a medical problem, so mention this to your medical provider. If you have a metallic taste in your mouth, avoid drinking from metal containers. Use plastic or wooden eating utensils. Choose foods with a lot of flavor or seasoning. Fool your taste buds by trying new foods. Suck on sugarless hard candies.

Day 199

Humor is mankind's greatest blessing.

—Mark Twain

Children laugh approximately 400 times a day; adults about 25. Although there has not been any research on the number of times HCV patients laugh during treatment, I'd guess it is a minus number. However, we can turn things around, just by making humor a priority.

Tip for Today: Make humor a regular part of your life. How about a hepatitis C cocktail hour? Before dinner, sit down with cheese and crackers, a tumbler of sparkling water, your ribavirin pills, and a joke book and keep reading until you have laughed at least twice. Don't turn on the news as this will undo the fun.

Day 200

Were the diver to think of the jaws of the shark, he would never lay hands on the precious pearl.

—Saadi Shirazi

You have been at this for 200 days, and this marks the fifth time you have endured a 40-day cycle. You have come a long way since the first injection. Use this landmark to evaluate where you are today in relation to your goals.

Tip for Today: Are you focusing on the shark or the pearl? If you are focusing on the shark, review your goals and reaffirm your resolve. If your eyes are on the pearl, savor the moment. Either way, you have made it through 200 days, proof that you can make it to the end.

Day 201

The best and most beautiful things in the world cannot be seen or even touched—they must be felt with the heart.

—Helen Keller

It's likely that you aren't feeling very attractive. Beauty may only be skin deep, but with hair loss, dry skin, and brittle nails, some of us wouldn't mind some superficial beauty. Those days will come back. For now try to see the beauty of your hard work. Your liver is probably looking especially gorgeous these days.

> **Tip for Today:** To reduce hair loss, use a wide-toothed comb. Limit brushing or combing to once a day; shampoo once or twice a week. Apply conditioner or detangling product after you wash. Use dry shampoo in place of regular shampoo. Sleep on satin pillow cases. Don't use devices that break the hair, such as clips, tight bands, or barrettes.

Day 202

Our attitude towards what has happened to us in life is the important thing to recognize. Once hopeless, my life is now hope-full, but it did not happen overnight. The last of human freedoms, to choose one's attitude in any given set of circumstances, is to choose one's own way.
—Viktor Frankl

Viktor Frankl, author of *Man's Search for Meaning*, was a psychiatrist and Holocaust survivor who lived through unimaginable horrors while still keeping a kind and generous spirit. I believe Frankl's words, but I am cautious when applying them to patients who are taking HCV medications. These drugs are potent and can affect the mind so dramatically that it may take more than sheer will to maintain a good attitude. However, it is still reasonable to strive for a good attitude, and in that there is freedom.

> **Tip for Today:** If you can't find pleasure in life, find it hard to get out of bed, or feel constantly down in the dumps, talk to your medical provider. You may be suffering from depression, and it is not too late to get help for this.

Day 203

If there is a way to do it better … find it.
—Thomas Edison

Fatigue is one of the most common side effects of HCV and its treatment. However, all too frequently, patients blame being tired on the medications. In fact, fatigue has many causes—some of which are easily fixed.

> **Tip for Today:** If you feel tired, be sure to rule out other causes of fatigue besides HCV medications. Here are a few questions to ask: Do you have insomnia? Do you have the symptoms of depression? Are you drinking enough liquids? Have you had lab tests to rule out anemia, diabetes, thyroid disease, and other conditions? Are you getting a little exercise every day? Are you eating a balanced diet, including regular meals? Are you experiencing a lot of stress? Have you discussed fatigue with your medical provider?

WEEK 30

Day 204

The key to your universe is that you can choose.
　　　　　　　　　　　　　　　　　—Frederick Frieseke

The raw truth is that in spite of the side effects and inconvenience, HCV treatment is a choice and a luxury. Many people are unable to do treatment, either because of health or financial reasons. As you pass the 30-week milestone, this is a good time to acknowledge your choice. There is every reason to believe you will make it to the end, but affirming your commitment may strengthen your resolve.

> **Tip for Today:** Use your key to the universe by choosing something that will help you weather the last few months of treatment. Find something that will capture your attention and keep your mind off side effects. Perhaps go to the movies or rent a video. You could get a subscription to a video rental service that sends DVDs directly to you or provides video streaming.

Day 205

In one hand I have a dream, and in the other I have an obstacle. Tell me, which one grabs your attention?
—Sir Henry Parkes

Despite the difficulty of HCV treatment, the majority of patients do not stop because of medication side effects. It helps to think of side effects as problems for which there are usually solutions. Keep your eye on the dream, and it is easier to get past the obstacle.

Tip for Today: One of the biggest obstacles that patients face during HCV treatment is itchy skin. Although usually not life threatening, skin disorders can create a lot of discord. If itching is a problem, discuss this with your medical provider, especially if you develop a rash. If your skin is dry, this may be causing or contributing to the problem. In addition to drinking lots of water and using body creams, put a humidifier in your bedroom and living areas. Wash clothes and sheets with baby laundry soap. Don't wear fabrics that are harsh on the skin, such as wool. More suggestions are listed in Appendix C: "Managing Skin Problems."

Day 206

I will never understand all the good that a simple smile can accomplish.
—Mother Teresa

Research tells us that smiling is good for our health. Smiling boosts the immune system, reduces stress, and lowers blood pressure. It also releases natural chemicals in the brain that help us feel better and cope with pain. Smiling has an infectious quality to it because when you smile, people smile back which makes you want to smile even more.

Tip for Today: The following exercise comes from Zen master, Thich Nhat Hanh: When you wake up, smile and breathe deeply three times. Repeat this as you go about your day.

Day 207

Surviving is important, but thriving is elegant.

—*Maya Angelou*

What ignites you and makes you feel alive? Even if you don't feel energetic, you can surround yourself with reminders of a joy-filled life. Perhaps you have photos of loved ones displayed where you can see them. Do you eat food that you enjoy? Is your bed comfortable? Do you have an attractive view of the world? Is there music in your life?

> **Tip for Today:** You can't thrive without food. Eat even if you have no appetite. To keep up your energy, try snacking at frequent intervals. Experiment with foods of varying textures. Perhaps you like cold crunchy items or foods such as soup or smoothies. Try foods you normally don't like to eat. Don't be surprised if you have acquired a taste for new foods or ones you previously disliked. If you can't think of a food to try, call a friend and ask for suggestions.

Day 208

I think pain is easiest to avoid by filling the days with distractions. ...

—*David Blaine*

When it comes to the use of distraction for pain, there are two opinions. One is to use distraction; the other is to avoid distraction. There is a place for each, whether the pain is physical or emotional. In my own life, initially, it helps me to acknowledge pain, to sit with it and to let it pass through me. I need to understand the nature of pain so I can determine how to confront it, and to ensure I don't make it worse. However, in the long term, it is best for me to keep my mind on other things so that pain doesn't become the focus of my life.

> **Tip for Today:** If you are uncomfortable, tired of treatment, having difficulty sleeping, or whatever, and you have discussed your condition with your medical provider, find something to distract you. Distraction works particularly well if you are tempted to dwell on how miserable you feel. My favorite distraction is listening to podcasts of humorous or compelling radio shows.

Day 209

Change the story and you change perception; change perception and you change the world.

—Jean Houston

What stories are you telling yourself? Is it a miserable one or a story filled with hope? What is your perception of HCV treatment? Are you a victim or a warrior? You get to decide what story to tell, and in your story, you can change the world.

> **Tip for Today:** One story that is hard to live with is gaining weight during HCV treatment. This may be due to a reduction in physical activity, an increase in calories, or the result of a medical problem, such as a thyroid abnormality. Discuss weight gain with your medical provider. At this point, you are probably not taking pills that must be taken with a high fat concentration, so you may cut back on the amount of fat you eat. Don't be hard on yourself about weight gain—that just makes matters worse.

Day 210

My life is shrinking during this time of treatment. My world is getting smaller and I am in great need of a God that is getting bigger!

—Kim Young

Today's quote is from a patient who figured out what she needed to endure treatment. Her life felt like it was getting smaller, and she knew she needed a way to make it bigger. If your life feels smaller, remember that the virus is shrinking too, and your liver is likely growing healthy, new, virus-free cells. Your life may feel smaller, but your future is growing.

> **Tip for Today:** The best way to keep your life large is to stay connected to people who will help you through treatment. There are some wonderful support groups on the Internet, such as groups on Facebook, Yahoo, and Google. People in the group will help expand your world and keep you tethered to hope.

WEEK 31

Day 211

To the mind that is still, the whole universe surrenders.

—Lao Tzu

Interferon has a way of activating a constant chatter in the brain. It feels like being held hostage by someone who won't shut up. It can be quite distracting, which at best sucks the pleasure out of life, and at worst draws our attention away from things that need our attention. Find ways to quiet your mind.

> **Tip for Today:** Meditation, the practice of quieting the mind, is a rewarding, profitable practice. Mindful meditation is particularly simple and the only way you can fail at it is to fail to do it. Mindful meditation is sometimes taught at hospitals, community colleges, and meditation centers. It can be self-taught with the aid of books, recordings, or the Internet.

Day 212

Change your thoughts and you change your world.

—Norman Vincent Peale

Language is a powerful tool that we can use to change our thoughts. Thoughts influence us—our choices, our health and how we perceive the world. For example, the word *patient* means "to endure pain or suffering" and "enduring trying circumstances with even temper." The words *patience* and *patient* share the same origin. As you head into the last quarter of your treatment, what kind of patient do you want to be—one who endures pain and suffering or one who endures trying circumstances with even temper?

> **Tip for Today:** Describe yourself with the most powerful language you can imagine:
> - I am a warrior.
> - I am a champion.
> - Treatment is easy, and my mood is light.

Day 213

Believe it can be done. When you believe something can be done, really believe, your mind will find the ways to do it. Believing a solution paves the way to solution.

—David Schwartz

Exhaustion can be a stubborn, relentless HCV-medication side effect, and may interfere with your ability to believe you can make it through HCV treatment. In *The Hepatitis C Help Book*, Misha Cohen and Robert Gish explain that Chinese medicine looks at fatigue as either a deficiency syndrome or as stagnant qi—the life force that runs through the body. Acupressure and other Chinese medicine techniques can help with fatigue and other treatment side effects, and is frequently covered by health insurance.

> **Tip for Today:** If you consult a Chinese medicine practitioner, find out about acupressure points for fatigue, so you can perform these at home. Confirm your understanding of these points by practicing them on yourself with the practitioner present.

Day 214

My liver swells with bile difficult to repress.

—Horace

In ancient times, the liver was considered to be the center of the body, similar to how we think of the heart. Anger was thought to destroy the liver. Science has revealed that constant anger can cause a cascade of destructive hormones and chemicals, which raises blood pressure and may injure the cardiovascular system. In short, anger is bad for the health.

> **Tip for Today:** Anger and rage can be controlled with anger-management tools. Meditation and biofeedback are two ways to control powerful emotions. However, HCV medications are so powerful that prescription drugs may offer a more effective way to manage this brief time of strong emotions. If you find yourself angry a great deal, talk to your medical provider.

Day 215

The first thing I do in the morning is to make my bed and while I am
making up my bed I am making up my mind as to what kind of a day
I am going to have.

—*Robert Frost*

Most of us get out of bed hoping for a good day. If side effects are particularly challenging, that good day may feel out of reach, particularly if you are continuing to work through treatment. If HCV treatment is interfering with your work, or if work is interfering with your ability to stay on treatment, make up your mind to protect your health and your job.

Tip for Today: Work is not always an all-or-nothing proposition. Consider the following:

- Work less, such as a four-day work week. You may want to schedule days off that are when you tend to have the most side effects.
- Adjust working hours to accommodate your best hours. You may feel great in the mornings and want to work 6 a.m. to 2 p.m. rather than 9 a.m. to 5 p.m.
- Telecommute. Some patients are able to work from home.
- Use your sick and vacation time to rest.

Day 216

Loneliness is proof that your innate search for connection is intact.

—*Martha Beck*

HCV treatment can be a lonely journey. The only people who seemed to understand me were those who had experience with treatment. I had contradictory feelings. On one hand, I struggled to stay strong and show that I could do anything. I rejected help from others. On the other hand, I was irritated that people didn't ask me how I was or notice how I felt. Now after many years of working with HCV patients, I see how invisible our illness is.

Tip for Today: Loneliness is uncomfortable. Maintain connection with the world. If you don't feel well or have trouble getting out, spend time reading HCV blogs or communicating with other people living with HCV. If you participate in an HCV group, your presence may help others. Giving support is a great remedy against isolation. A list of blogs may be found in the Resources guide at the back of this book, and you should also look at the entries under "Support Groups" or "Storytelling."

Day 217

If you want to test your memory, try to recall what you were worrying about one year ago today.

—Rotarian

Our ability to remember deteriorates during HCV treatment with one notable exception—we can't seem to forget things that bother us. Wouldn't it be wonderful if we could forget those things too? It's quite likely that a year from now you won't remember most of today's problems.

Tip for Today: You may have issues, bills, or other details that need attention or resolution. If your memory seems unreliable, get in the habit of recording details. Every time you call your insurance company, medical office, or other type of business, keep notes of dates, names, and issues that you discussed. If you have e-mail records, save these too. Keep notes in one central location.

WEEK 32

Day 218

You don't have to cook fancy or complicated masterpieces—just good food from fresh ingredients.

—Julia Child

The monotony of treatment can steal the pleasure out of eating. However, eating at regular intervals is essential, because the body will not function without sufficient fuel. A simple diet consisting of easily prepared foods will help you sustain your energy without wiping out your available reserves.

> **Tip for Today:** When you can, eat your favorite fresh ingredients. However, there may be days when you are too tired to shop or cook, so keep a supply of nutritious snacks that are simple to prepare. Stock up on healthy muffins, applesauce, yogurt, soup, granola bars, string cheese, whole grain waffles, nuts, trail mix, or cereal. Some patients find it easy to consume nutritional drinks, such as powdered instant breakfast, Ensure, or similar products from their local health food store.

Day 219

Do not undervalue the headache. While it is at its sharpest it seems a bad investment; but when relief begins, the unexpired remainder is worth $4 a minute.

—*Mark Twain*

Sometimes the way through pain is to find ways to endure it, particularly chronic, tolerable pain. Mark Twain endured a lot of pain in his life, and humor was one of the tools he used to help him through the hard times. Humor increases endorphins and can relieve discomfort.

> **Tip for Today:** In addition to humor, aromatherapy may help with headaches. Use this remedy cautiously as odors can trigger headaches or nausea. Lavender, peppermint, eucalyptus, or rosemary is recommended to soothe headaches. The remedy that helped my treatment-related headaches was to relax in a dark room and cover my forehead and eyes with a small silk pillow filled with fresh lavender. You can experiment with essential oils rubbed into the temples, forehead, or base of the skull.

Day 220

The art of love ... is largely the art of persistence.

—*Albert Ellis*

Persistence may be vital to the art of love, but open and honest communication is also critical for the health of a relationship. If there is a sexual problem and you aren't discussing it, it's like the proverbial elephant in the room that no one says anything about. If you are reluctant to discuss relationship problems with your partner, at least acknowledge the problems. You may say that these issues are hard to discuss while you are taking HCV medications, and that you appreciate your partner's patience.

> **Tip for Today:** If your sex life has fallen by the wayside, explore new ways to meet your partner's needs. If sexual intercourse is a problem, find other ways to be intimate. Experiment with massage or a candlelit evening at home watching a romantic movie. There are many ways to spice up life when it feels dull. If this feels like it is too much for you to undertake, ask your partner to take the initiative.

Day 221

What I need is someone who will make me do what I can.

—Ralph Waldo Emerson

HCV treatment can be like a relationship; after awhile it is easy to get complacent. At this point, it is likely that you are spending less time researching how to manage side effects, perhaps hoping you can just put up with everything until the end. Although your medical provider is the "go to" authority for side effect management, it may be worth investing a little time gathering tips to relieve some of your most annoying complaints.

> **Tip for Today:** Pharmaceutical companies provide excellent support and information for consumers. They can send information, or you can review what they provide on the Internet. Call the pharmacy support lines to get more information or to talk to a nurse about something specific.

Day 222

When we are no longer able to change a situation, we are challenged to change ourselves.

—Viktor Frankl

As HCV treatment continues to hammer on you, it can be tempting to try complementary and alternative medicine. Herbs and other dietary supplements are powerful ways to manage health problems, but they can also be dangerous. Some people think that because herbs are natural that means they are safe. Strychnine and snake venom are natural but certainly aren't safe.

> **Tip for Today:** Some herbs use the same metabolic pathways that HCV medications use, increasing the risk of having too much or too little either of the HCV drug or the supplement. As mentioned earlier, if you are taking an HCV protease inhibitor, do not take St. John's wort. If you are interested in herbs and supplements, talk to your medical provider first. Acupressure and healing arts that don't use supplementation are generally safe.

Day 223

Anything one man can imagine, other men can make real.
—Jules Verne

Success and visualization often go hand in hand. When asked what the secret to their success was, many accomplished people say they visualized winning or pictured their future self. Vision boards are used as motivational tools in business settings as well as for personal growth. When you began treatment, even if you weren't conscious of it, you probably visualized making it through and being free of HCV. If you hadn't pictured this, you probably would not have started on this path in the first place.

> **Tip for Today:** Visualization is a powerful tool you can use to help you reach the finish line. In your mind's eye, picture an effortless treatment, free of side effects. Visualize feeling energetic and strong. Imagine your doctor telling you that you are cured of hepatitis C.

Day 224

The only difference between a rut and a grave is their dimensions.
—Ellen Glasgow

You may feel like you are in a bit of a rut. After all, you have been at this treatment for more than seven months. If you are feeling tired of it all, find ways to distract yourself from the rut you're in. Take comfort in the fact that you are two-thirds of the way through treatment.

> **Tip for Today:** Stir up your life by stepping past your comfort zone. Go to a museum or zoo, where you can walk and sit. Visit a park that has plenty of benches. Turn off the TV, sit, and stare out the window. Go to the library and borrow an audio book or music. Buy yourself some flowers or a new gadget. Steer your life out of the rut.

WEEK 33

Day 225

A positive attitude and a sense of humor go together like biscuits and gravy.

—Dolly Parton

Here is the hepatitis C version of Dolly Parton's saying: A negative attitude and no sense of humor go with interferon and ribavirin. However, don't let that stop you from finding something to laugh at, especially if you are laughing at yourself.

> **Tip for Today:** Humor is a recognized way of coping with difficulty. However, you may have days when you need more than a good laugh. Try taking a holiday from your problems. Make a list of everything that annoys you and declare that you are taking a vacation day from these irritants. To help you get started, here are a few things from my list: computers, telephone solicitors, well-meaning family members, the news, and people who let their dogs run loose.

Day 226

Fall seven times, stand up eight.

—Japanese Proverb

Although you are getting close to the end of treatment, don't stop looking for ways to manage side effects. It's all too easy to give up and just try to muscle through it all, but you really don't have to. If you discover a new way to manage a side effect and get some benefit, does it really matter that this occurred late in your treatment?

Tip for Today: If you live in a dry climate, your skin may feel like beef jerky. For extreme dryness, rub A & D ointment or petroleum jelly between your hands and then apply a light layer over damp skin immediately following bathing. At bedtime, apply a thin layer of A & D or petroleum jelly to your hands, and cover with cotton gloves to protect bed linens.

Day 227

Life is difficult, it is true, a struggle from minute to minute ... but the struggle itself is thrilling.

—Etty Hillesum

This wisdom was written by Etty Hillesum, a 27-year-old Jewish woman who lived in Amsterdam under Nazi occupation. Her journals and letters are remarkable, particularly because her passion for life is so intense. While en route from the Westerbork transit camp in Holland to a death camp at Auschwitz in Poland, she threw a card out of the train. Found by farmers, the card said, "We left the camp singing." With death squarely in front of her, she found strength; with life in front of you, may you also find strength.

Tip for Today: Find joy today even if you think there is nothing to be happy about. If you can't sing, listen to music. Look at photographs or art. Read the latest sports news. Step outside and breathe in the fresh air. Call someone who is having a hard time.

Day 228

One doesn't discover new lands without consenting to lose sight of the shore for a very long time.

—André Gide

It may feel as if you have been separated from yourself for so long that you can't remember what healthy felt like. During hard times, hold fast to those things that will heal you, such as rest, good food, support, meditation, humor, and staying active. Avoid drugs and alcohol, as these will undo your tremendous efforts.

> **Tip for Today:** HCV treatment may bring up cravings or aggravate substance abuse problems. If you are in a recovery program, increase your efforts to stay clean and sober. If you don't have support, get it. If you aren't in a recovery program, but feel as if you may drink or use drugs, get professional help and/or attend a recovery group.

Day 229

The only tired I was, was tired of giving in.
—Rosa Parks

It can be tempting to give up and just say, "I am sick." But are you really? Undoubtedly you feel sick, but aren't you in fact building health? The moment you started HCV treatment, you took action to stop being sick and start being well.

> **Tip for Today:** How physically active are you? Are you going for regular walks or engaging in activities that keep you moving, limber, and strong? This is important. If you aren't moving much, incorporate light activity in small increments into your day. There are exercises for all ranges of people who have difficulty staying active, from couch potatoes to those with serious diseases. Look for suggestions on the Internet and at your local library, or talk to your medical provider.

Day 230

Gratitude is so close to the bone of life, pure and true, that it instantly stops the rational mind, and all its planning and plotting.
—Regina Sara Ryan

It is virtually impossible to feel grateful and irritable at the same time. It may feel like a huge leap to get from a bad mood to a grateful one, but it is a leap where you only risk feeling wonderful. Few things lift the spirit as effectively as gratitude.

> **Tip for Today:** If you are feeling down, irritable, or filled with self-pity, try this: Write down at least five things for which you are grateful. If you are in an especially bad mood, you may have to fake it, and say things such as "I am grateful I didn't commit homicide today." Keep a gratitude journal and write in it every day.

Day 231

Variety is the spice of life.

—American Proverb

I am not saying anything you don't already know when I mention that treatment can get tedious. If you are feeling as if you are just marking time, explore ways to bring pleasure and change into your daily routine. Yes, you are marking time, but wouldn't you rather it passed pleasurably?

Tip for Today: If you are getting bored with water, try drinking tea. There are so many varieties of tea that you could try a different one every day and never run out of things to try. Herbal tea may soothe an upset stomach, clear congestion, or help with a headache. Some teas, such as green and black, have caffeine, so these are better consumed earlier in the day. Tea can be served with honey, mint, or lemon, as well as hot or cold.

WEEK 34

Day 232

Birds learn how to fly, never knowing where flight will take them.

—Mark Nepo

HCV treatment is like learning how to fly. When you start, you aren't sure if you will stay aloft. You may have a destination, but in fact, you are flying around in unknown territory for the entire time. You are buffeted by storms, and in the end you may not reach the place you intended to land.

Tip for Today: If you can, for one day, or one hour, or one minute, allow yourself to be in flight, without thoughts of where you would rather be. Focus on your body that has carried you these many months. Look around at your surroundings. Marvel at the fact that you have stayed aloft thus far.

Day 233

If you light a lamp for someone else it will also brighten your path.

—Buddha

When we are in the throes of the side effects from HCV antiviral medications, helping others isn't something we think about doing. The paradox is that sometimes this is exactly what we need to consider; when we help someone else, we are lifted out of our own misery.

Tip for Today: Find a small way to help another. Send an encouraging note, e-mail, or text message. Call someone who is having a bad time. Go for a short walk and pick up some trash—but be careful if dizziness is a problem. Put a quarter into an expired parking meter. Brighten someone else's life, and yours will feel brighter too.

Day 234

The body is consuming energy when tense, and restoring energy when it is relaxed.

—Ronnie Lott

Stress and worry put constant tension on the muscles. Not only does this use up valuable energy, it restricts blood flow to surrounding tissue. Right now you don't have extra energy to spare. Learn to relax, and you will find residual power that you can call on to help you through the day.

Tip for Today: Throughout the day, find time to relax and clear you head. Sit in a quiet place, close your eyes and take 10 slow, deep breaths. Notice any unusually tight or sore spots in your body, and imagine breathing into those places. Do this even if you don't feel like it, aiming for two or more times daily.

Day 235

When the well is dry, they know the worth of the water.

—Benjamin Franklin

You may be getting used to the side effects of treatment, but just because you are used to them doesn't mean that you shouldn't look for ways to alleviate them. I have been helping people manage HCV treatment side effects since 1998, and I am still learning new tips.

Tip for Today: Manufacturers of dry mouth remedies are constantly introducing new products. Early in treatment, you may have tried your local drugstore or online pharmacy, looking for relief from dry mouth. If you are bothered by constant dry mouth, check to see if there are any new products to help with this. Ask your dentist for free samples of products.

Day 236

The voyage of the best ship is a zigzag line of a hundred tacks.
—*Ralph Waldo Emerson*

Hepatitis C treatment may feel like going from one side effect to the next, like one of those awful stories that goes, "I thought that was bad, not realizing what would happen next." In truth, HCV treatment is more like a sailboat zigzagging in the wind, looking for the safest way to sail home. The good news is that the voyage doesn't last forever.

Tip for Today: If you are feeling weary of HCV treatment and its side effects, focus on a few facts:
1. There is an end to treatment.
2. You are more than two-thirds of the way through treatment.
3. As uncomfortable as treatment is, it is helping your liver, your life, and your future.

Day 237

Some people have a wonderful capacity to appreciate again and again, freshly and naively, the basic goods of life, with awe, pleasure, wonder, and even ecstasy.
—*Abraham H. Maslow*

Even under the best of circumstances, the ability to appreciate the beauty and wonder of life is a precious gift. HCV treatment may feel more like daily drudgery rather than awe or ecstasy. However, it is possible to find pleasure during treatment. Look for wonder in simple things, such as food, nature, being with a pet, or when listening to favorite music.

Tip for Today: Food is one of life's basic pleasures, and it can be frustrating if you lose the joy of eating. Experiment with foods you may not regularly choose. Go to a deli or health food store and try something new. If you are too tired to get out of your car, most fast food establishments have a selection of nutritious foods, such as fruit smoothies. If you don't want to leave the house, ask a friend to surprise you with something delicious.

Day 238

We are what we think. All that we are rises with our thoughts. With our thoughts, we make the world.

—Buddha

I believe in the power of positive thinking. However, when I was on HCV treatment, if someone told me to "just think positive," I would have probably flown off the handle. Telling people on mind-altering interferon to "think positive" is like telling a person with no legs to "get up and walk." Perhaps it is best to set the intention to have a positive attitude, rather than focusing on the results. However, it is always worth aiming high.

Tip for Today: Despite the mind's rebellious qualities during HCV treatment, affirmative thoughts do work. The most important tool to use is acceptance. Accept whatever thoughts float by, and then let them continue to pass until they drop off the horizon of your mind. Chastising yourself for negative thinking just creates more negative thinking, so let self-critical thoughts fly by as if they were just passing through the area without encouraging them to stop and spend the night.

WEEK 35

Day 239

Man needs difficulties; they are necessary for health.

—Carl Gustav Jung

How could the difficulty of living with HCV and going through treatment be necessary for health? You might not find the answer to this question for a long time, but one day this journey will show its purpose and may help you in amazing ways.

> **Tip for Today:** Difficulties may be a necessary part of health, but problems are not a test of endurance. Take a moment to perform a mini-assessment of your body. Is anything bothering you that you haven't mentioned to your medical provider? Perhaps you haven't said anything because you don't want to trouble anyone. However, helping you is your provider's job. If you have questions, call your medical provider's office, and let an expert decide if you need to be seen. You pay for this expertise, so you might as well use it.

Day 240

A jug fills drop by drop.

—*Buddha*

Think about an empty jug and how long it would take to fill it drop by drop. That's essentially where you started 240 days ago. Day by day, pill by pill, you got here, and now there are less than 100 days ahead. Your jug is almost full.

> **Tip for Today:** This is the sixth 40-day segment through the trials and tribulations of treatment. Review your goals. What do you need to help you through to the end? Although there are less than 100 days left, you still have some distance to travel. Figure out what you need and recommit yourself to your goals.

Day 241

Anger is a brief lunacy.

—*Horace*

Anger, resentment, and rage may feel like an unwanted excursion into insanity. These powerful emotions hurt us and those around us. It is common to feel irritable, particularly after months of relentless side effects. However, rage is an extreme form of this and may require medical intervention. Do not let yourself get carried to this extreme.

Tip for Today: If you feel angry, try to figure out the cause. Are you hungry, tired, depressed, or overworked? Are you just tired of treatment and the side effects? Talk to your medical provider to see if you need help with stress reduction, anger management, or medication; if you are already taking medication perhaps an increase in dosage will help.

Day 242

If I had a party to attend and didn't want to be there, I would play the part of someone who was having a lovely time.

—*Shirley MacLaine*

HCV treatment often feels like an event that one does not want to attend. This time is fraught with difficulties, but fighting it makes the situation worse. The way of nonresistance is the easier path.

Tip for Today: Acceptance is a powerful tool. When acceptance is difficult to embrace, "acting as if" may help get you there. Try acting as if you feel good, and that HCV treatment is easy. When life is difficult, pretend for just one hour that you are perfectly fine and enjoying life.

Day 243

Sameness is the mother of disgust, variety the cure.

—*Francesco Petrarch*

Today's quote may not be true all the time, but when boredom sets in, variety is a pleasant solution. The closer you get to the finish line, the harder it is to find ways to keep life interesting. You don't have to grit your teeth and just make it through—try to find some pleasure in these last few months.

> **Tip for Today:** If you are tired of drinking water and other beverages, eat foods that have high water content. Watermelon, cantaloupes, oranges, and popsicles are high in water. Alternatively, start your day with a large jug of water. Add mint, cucumber, or fruit to it, and put it in the refrigerator. Experiment with various combinations to flavor your water.

Day 244

People often say that motivation doesn't last. Well, neither does bathing —that's why we recommend it daily.

—*Zig Ziglar*

Every day is a new day, whether you are on treatment or not. Every day you get to figure out how to make it through this journey. It is best to use a shot of inspiration and motivation from somewhere, since like most people going through HCV treatment, you may need some help to get through difficult times.

> **Tip for Today:** Cultivate ways to stay motivated. Talk to people who support you. Read inspirational blogs, books, and articles. Remember why you are doing this treatment.

Day 245

If you don't do what's best for your body, you're the one who comes up on the short end.

—*Julius Erving*

It can be difficult to take care of yourself during HCV treatment. You may just want to curl up in bed, turn the lights off, and wait until this entire ordeal is over. However, the ordeal is best endured if you take care of your basic needs, such as doing light to moderate exercise, eating healthy foods, and living a life that balances rest and activity.

Tip for Today: From time to time, ask yourself what you need most. Are you staying active? Getting enough sleep? Are you staying in touch with friends and other important people in your life? Are you eating healthy food? How is your spirit? Is there any fun in your life? Address any areas where you may be feeling out of balance.

WEEK 36

Day 246

Pain has its reasons, pleasure is totally indifferent.

—*Francis Picabia*

It can be tempting to think that every symptom is caused by HCV treatment. Now that you have completed three-quarters of your peginterferon injections, you may tell yourself that certain problems can wait until you are done with treatment, hoping these will go away. However, not everything is caused by HCV medications, and if there is another cause, you may miss the chance to fix a small problem before it turns into a bigger one. When we blame everything on HCV treatment, a door of opportunity may slam shut—a door that could lead to relief.

Tip for Today: Do you have any medical problems that haven't been discussed with your medical provider? If so, consider contacting him or her, by e-mail, phone, or by making an appointment.

Day 247

The real test of friendship is: can you literally do nothing with the other person? Can you enjoy those moments of life that are utterly simple?

—*Eugene Kennedy*

Hepatitis C treatment is a trial that no one should endure alone. We can get mired in despair and lose our bearings. It may be difficult to explain to someone what HCV treatment feels like, but even if we can't, we can still sit with a friend and enjoy life's simple pleasures.

Tip for Today: Do you have a friend who cares for you without needing explanations? Do you have a friend to whom you can say anything and know you will be heard? If you were talking with a friend, what would you say is your biggest concern right now? If you haven't said this aloud to anyone, be sure you do. In the long run, it is better to air our problems.

Day 248

I merely took the energy it takes to pout and wrote some blues.
—Duke Ellington

The side effects from HCV treatment are real, and wishing them away is unlikely to make much of an impact. However, we don't have to feel sorry for ourselves. Self-pity just takes more energy—more than we can spare.

Tip for Today: If you are feeling self-pity, find some way to channel this. Help another, go to an HCV group, dig in the garden, and write a poem—anything to step outside of yourself. Of course, if you are a songwriter, perhaps "The Interferon Blues" will make it to the top of the charts.

Day 249

Alone I was feeling the heat of dying. But once voicing my pain in a circle of others on the same path, my heart relaxed back into the light of living.
—Mark Nepo

In *The Book of Awakening*, Nepo describes what happens when we suffer alone, comparing it to what happens when light is confined—it turns to heat. When we isolate ourselves with harsh thoughts, it is similar to building a fire in a confined space. If left too long, it is like being burned alive. We can't find our way back out if the light that shows the way is suffocated.

> **Tip for Today:** Are there any thoughts that you keep confined, thoughts that are slowly burning away at your peace of mind or suffocating you? If so, find a way to release them, such as by talking to a trusted friend or by writing down what is going on, and leaving it alone for a while. Step out of isolation into the cool light of hope.

Day 250

If we had no winter, the spring would not be so pleasant; if we did not sometimes taste of adversity, prosperity would not be so welcome.
—Anne Bradstreet

When I was at my lowest point in treatment, I kept thinking about the fact that summer would eventually arrive, and with it came watermelons. The promise of watermelons kept me going, and I ate that juicy fruit every day it was in season. I completed treatment just as watermelons were going out of season.

> **Tip for Today:** What do you love about life? What brings you joy? Even if you have not felt joy in a while, are you able to wrap your memory around those things in life that lifted your heart and called you to go through HCV treatment so you could live longer and better? Write these down so, in case you forget, you have reminders to help you stay on course.

Day 251

Health is not simply the absence of sickness.
—Hannah Green

Health is an attitude. It is also a commitment. During HCV treatment, you may not feel healthy, but keep in mind that even when you are experiencing side effects you are helping your liver and building health.

Tip for Today: You are the healthcare consumer; your body belongs to you. When you see your medical provider, take control of the appointment by being prepared. Write down everything in advance of your appointment, including questions and a prioritized list of issues you want to address.

Day 252

Part of the happiness of life consists not in fighting battles, but in avoiding them. A masterly retreat is in itself a victory.
—*Norman Vincent Peale*

Hepatitis C treatment is sometimes called "fighting the dragon." It is an apt metaphor, given how difficult treatment is. The fight is hardest towards the end, when the drugs are causing many side effects and the finish line seems so far away. Rather than continuing to fight, consider surrendering to the process. Surrendering is not quitting—it is simply not fighting. When you stop fighting, it shifts the focus off the struggle, making it easier to see other options.

Tip for Today: Are you fighting treatment? If so, drop your weapons and rest for a bit. Imagine that the wind is carrying you and will take you to a soft landing in about 12 weeks. One more suggestion: celebrate crossing the three-quarter milestone. Your soft landing is within reach.

6

●●●●●●●

Readings for the Final 12 Weeks

Note: In extremely rare instances, your medical provider may prescribe more than 48 weeks of treatment. If this happens, hold off reading this chapter until your treatment end date is 12 weeks away. Sometimes the decision to extend treatment is made late in the game, so stop wherever you are in the book, and fill in with extra daily readings found in any portion of this book that you have not read, or re-read entries that you found helpful. Expanded treatment can be discouraging news; try your best to stay positive and focused on taking care of yourself.

THE FINAL TWELVE WEEKS

Countdown: 84 days left

Don't watch the clock; do what it does. Keep going.
—Samuel Levenson

Congratulations! More of your treatment is behind you than ahead of you. Many patients shift into a countdown mode after passing this milestone. This is normal. However, sometimes the desire to be done bestows heaviness rather than lightness. Celebrate your success, but stay in the present as much as possible. Successful completion of HCV treatment rests on taking care of yourself today.

Tip for Today: If you want to count treatment days, count those that are over, along with those that are left. Your pile of days will look much bigger from this perspective. If your treatment length is 24 weeks, today is the 85th day. If you are on a full 48-week plan, you are on day 253. Either way, today is the most important day.

Countdown: 83 days left

It is easier to act your way into a new way of thinking than to think your way into a new way of acting.

—Alcoholics Anonymous

Fatigue is a common side effect of HCV treatment. Although painless, exhaustion can feel paralyzing, robbing you of your ability to function. We know that HCV medications cause fatigue; however, multiple studies suggest that positive thinking may relieve tiredness. Research supports the use of affirmations, along with the avoidance of negative statements to boost the perception of less exhaustion. In other words, those who focus on fatigue and reinforce this with negative self-talk report feeling more tired than those who tell themselves that they have plenty of energy.

Tip for Today: Say affirmations to yourself, and be on the lookout for negative self-talk. If you notice yourself saying, "I feel tired," try different words, such as, "I feel my energy coming back" or "I will rest for a few minutes and then get up feeling refreshed and recharged."

Countdown: 82 days left

We can be sure that the greatest hope for maintaining equilibrium in the face of any situation rests within ourselves.

—Francis J. Braceland

Now that you are nearing the end of HCV treatment, you may be longing for endurance rather than equilibrium. However, endurance requires a certain amount of balance; otherwise we fall down. Everything you need is inside of you.

Tip for Today: This qigong exercise is purported to restore balance to the internal organs. Stand in the qigong position discussed on Day 93 or sit in the one presented on Day 178. Raise your arms slowly until your hands are over your head. Turn palms up, reaching toward the sky. When arms are straight, but not strained, hold for a moment; then gently lower hands to the top of your head. Breathe, and then extend arms upward again. Do this eight times; fewer if you feel tired.

Countdown: 81 days left

Fake feeling good.... You're going to have to learn to fake cheerfulness. Believe it or not, eventually that effort will pay off: you'll actually start feeling happier.

—Jean Bach

It is strange, but acting as if you feel good can actually improve the way you perceive things. It certainly doesn't hurt to try this, as you have nothing to lose except your misery.

Tip for Today: If hair loss is causing you grief, try a new hair style. Hats are fashionable for men and women, and they can transform a bad hair day. A wig or hairpiece is another way to lift your spirits. When you are done with treatment, your hair will start getting thicker in about three months. However, it will be a while until the new growth reaches the length you desire, so experiment with styles or hats until your hair returns.

Countdown: 80 days left

Hold a true friend with both hands.

—Nigerian Proverb

You may not feel like socializing, but HCV treatment is easier to do when you aren't isolated. A good friend is like a life preserver, keeping us buoyant when the waves are most threatening. When was the last time you spent time with a friend?

Tip for Today: Have a tea party, but not one of those frilly, delicate porcelain affairs. Invite friends to bring their favorite teas for you to try during your treatment. Boil some water, set out some mugs, and sample one or two cups of tea. If you aren't feeling up to this, ask them to bring their own mugs or to just give you the tea. While you are at it, ask them to bring some cookies. If you don't like tea, have a juice party.

Countdown: 79 days left

It is easier to find men who will volunteer to die, than to find those who are willing to endure pain with patience.

—Julius Caesar

Toward the end of my HCV treatment, if someone told me to be patient, especially regarding pain, I might have gone ballistic. I am not going to tell you to be patient, but I will tell you that this all will pass. You will get your life back. Do everything you can to make it safely to the finish line.

Tip for Today: Patience is a rare quality in those who suffer pain. If you have a headache, other ache, or problem that is starting to get to you, but not severe enough to require urgent medical attention, find a quiet, dark place to lie down. Let your body sink into the mattress. Starting with your feet, imagine that each muscle is letting go and for that moment, leave your cares outside of the room. If thoughts start to intrude, tell yourself that you can think about them later. Do this every time you find yourself having such thoughts, even if they recur a thousand times. Spend as much time as you need to recover some strength and patience.

Countdown: 78 days left

A danger half seen is half avoided.

—Cheyenne Proverb

HCV treatment probably feels routine at this point. You may be handling it well, but there is always room to learn better ways to manage side effects. With the end of treatment so close, this is not the time to become complacent.

> **Tip for Today:** Take some time to review information about HCV treatment. In particular, read up on side effect management tips. You may pick up some new information to make it easier during these last weeks. If you belong to an HCV group, ask others to share tips.

THE FINAL ELEVEN WEEKS

Countdown: 77 days left

Some days there won't be a song in your heart. Sing anyway.
—Emory Austin

Few patients sing their way through the last part of treatment. At this juncture you are probably resting more than you did in the beginning of treatment. It is crucial that you continue to eat and drink enough, as fuel and hydration are necessary for health. Encourage yourself to do those things that are good for you, even if you don't want to do them. You are almost done with treatment; taking care of yourself today is an investment in your future.

> **Tip for Today:** Even if you don't feel like eating, do it anyway. Make an honest assessment of your food and fluid intake. If you aren't taking in sufficient fluids and nutrients, make a contract with yourself to eat and drink liquids even if you don't feel like it. Be especially diligent about drinking water and other fluids. Set a goal, write it down, follow it, and evaluate your progress each week.

Countdown: 76 days left

Every day is a good day.
—Zen Proverb

If you think you are having a bad day, bear in mind that it is a privilege to be able to do HCV treatment, since many people cannot afford it. You are giving your liver a huge gift, and you have proven yourself to be a brave person. Any day spent with a beating heart is a good day.

Tip for Today: Your mind can be a powerful ally if you use it well. Just for today, tell yourself and everyone else you are having a good day, even if you feel lousy. You don't need to convince yourself of the quality of the day; just claim that it is a good one, even if it feels artificial.

Countdown: 75 days left

He who laughs, lasts!

—*Mary Pettibone Poole*

The best way I can describe HCV treatment to those who haven't gone through it is to inject a little humor. It's like being at a high altitude, except the view is lousy. You feel tired and lethargic. Your skin is dry; your mouth is sore. You have a headache, you are breathless, and everything hurts. When you reach the summit, there won't be any photos, and when you are done with the climb, you can't have champagne. Despite it all, it is worth it, and you are worth it.

Tip for Today: Describe your experience of treatment to someone who doesn't have HCV or to someone who has gone through HCV treatment. Try to tell it with some humor.

Countdown: 74 days left

Sometimes a wound is the place where we encounter life for the first time, where we come to know its powers and its ways. Wounded, we may find a wisdom that will enable us to live better than any knowledge, and glimpse a view of ourselves and of life that is both true and unexpected.

—*Rachel Naomi Remen*

HCV treatment is a time when we become quite acquainted with our deepest wounds. We have two choices: (a) practice patience and allow healing to take place, (b) keep ripping off the scabs and stay in pain. The capacity to heal is in our hands.

> **Tip for Today:** Cuts, scrapes, rashes, and other injuries to the skin take longer to heal during HCV treatment. This is standard. Signs of infection, such as redness, swelling, pus, or pain are not normal and need medical attention. Dry skin takes longer to heal, so remember to use creams and moisturizers.

Countdown: 73 days left

When angry, count four; when very angry, swear.

—Mark Twain

Scientists have studied people who cuss when responding to pain. Those who let loose swear words are less sensitive to pain and are able to endure discomfort for longer durations. Now that is one study that I would not want to volunteer for. What if I was put in the group that had to endure pain without swearing? In fact, the moment I was told I would have to endure pain, I'd probably say, "hell no" before the study even got started.

> **Tip for Today:** If swearing isn't against your moral code, then go ahead and say those four-letter words after you stub a toe or slam a finger in the door. It's probably best not to do this in public. Although it is good to let our feelings out, don't direct your anger toward others. Take action to let go of your feelings and move on.

Countdown: 72 days left

Every time you express gratitude or compassion for any aspect of your-self or someone else, you breathe life in.

—Mariah Fenton Gladis

The practice of gratitude is a potent tool that can chase away pain and dark moods. Even when one does not feel grateful, practicing it can have a powerful effect on us and those around us.

> **Tip for Today:** A gratitude practice can bestow multiple benefits. Not only does it elevate the mood, but it also can help with insomnia. If you are having trouble falling asleep, name everything for which you are thankful. Here is one to get you started, "I am grateful for my bed and pillow."

Countdown: 71 days left

Health is the consummation of a love affair of all the organs of the body.
— *Plato*

Good health includes sex, and when interest in this is diminished because of HCV treatment, it can feel like a great loss. This loss may be deeper for your sexual partner, and may lead to discord between you both. Be sure to tell your partner how much you care about him or her.

> **Tip for Today:** If you don't feel like having sex, perhaps you can find ways to meet your partner's needs. Encourage your partner to be open about what these needs might be. Remember that the most powerful sexual organ is the brain. Your brain might not be functioning well, so perhaps your partner can suggest ways to get through this temporary challenge.

THE FINAL TEN WEEKS

Countdown: 70 days left

I've learned from experience that the greater part of our happiness or misery depends on our dispositions and not on our circumstances.
— *Martha Washington*

During the course of HCV treatment, you may sometimes feel that you have a better chance of climbing a mountain than changing your disposition. However, even prisoners of war and other victims of horrendous circumstances have found ways to keep their spirits from flagging. It all comes down to attitude. The first step is willingness.

> **Tip for Today:** One way to improve a bad attitude is with affirmations. Throughout the day, repeat positive phrases to yourself, especially when you encounter negative thoughts. Here are a few to try:
> - My body is healing.
> - I am strong.
> - I am alive and well.
> - Every cell in my body vibrates with energy.
> - I am grateful and content.

Countdown: 69 days left

Breathe in, breathe out. Forget this and enlightenment is unattainable.
—Author unknown

Throughout treatment, you may have noticed an unfriendly, disagreeable voice in your head, telling you all sorts of negative or frightening things. These thoughts may be about how others are acting, or about your own ability to make it through treatment. This internal voice may sound overwhelmed, claiming that life is impossible. In those moments, when the hold on life is fragile, the goal may simply be to survive the day. The secret to survival may be condensed to this single practice, "Breathe in, breathe out."

Tip for Today: Breathe in, breathe out. Keep repeating.

Countdown: 68 days left

Sleep is the golden chain that ties health and our bodies together.
—Thomas Dekker

If you are having problems with fatigue, don't assume that there is nothing you can do about this just because you've been taking HCV medications for awhile. Look at the quality and amount of your sleep. Are you sleeping enough? Do you wake up frequently? If so, is something waking you up, such as noise, the temperature of the room, or frequent trips to the bathroom? Is pain waking you up? Pets in the bedroom or a snoring partner are sleep interrupters. Be sure to discuss sleep problems with your medical provider, especially if pain is contributing to the problem.

Tip for Today: Experiment with ways to improve your sleep. Don't drink too many liquids close to bedtime. If pets must sleep in your room, reduce noise by removing their collars. Keep your room cool but your body warm. If your partner is snoring, he or she may need medical help. In the meantime, try earplugs or separate rooms. If sleep remains elusive, talk to your medical provider about sleep medication.

Countdown: 67 days left

When the heart grieves over what is lost, the spirit rejoices over what is left.

—Sufi Proverb

These days you may not feel as if there is much left that hasn't been destroyed by HCV treatment. However, if you have one strand of hair left, can breathe, walk, see, and hear, you have plenty to rejoice over. The fact that your body is strong enough to carry you this distance is evidence that you still have much in your life.

> **Tip for Today:** Make a list of the good things you have in your life. If you can't think of anything, perhaps you are depressed and need to talk to your medical provider about this. If you can make a list but don't want to, and you are thinking of ripping up this book and mailing it to me in tiny shreds, hang in there; this will pass.

Countdown: 66 days left

I think the next best thing to solving a problem is finding some humor in it.

—Frank A. Clark

Are you feeling as if you are losing your mind? Is brain fog getting you down? Although HCV treatment feels dreadful at times, it has qualities that make it ripe for comic relief. And in that, laughter makes treatment bearable.

> **Tip for Today:** Humor helped me tolerate frustrating moments. When I couldn't remember a word, I claimed I had Hepheimer's. When I lost my temper, it was because of Riberette's syndrome. I blamed my moods on mentalpause. I was not poking fun at Alzheimer's, Tourette's, or menopause—I was laughing at myself. Look for witty or absurd ways to describe your experiences.

Countdown: 65 days left

The human spirit cannot be paralyzed. If you are breathing, you can dream.

—Mike Brown

It can be hard to remember what it felt like before HCV treatment; harder still to imagine what it will be like when you are finished and the medications' side effects have worn off. Still, you are breathing and you are alive. Don't forget to dream, and while you are at it, dream big. You are the one who determines the size and contents of your dreams.

> **Tip for Today:** While you are daydreaming, spice up your breath and your life by chewing or sucking on fresh parsley or anise seeds. Cinnamon or mint gum will help dry mouth and breath. For variety, chew sugarless bubble gum or one of the dessert-flavored gums, such as apple pie or strawberry shortcake.

Countdown: 64 days left

Attention to health is life's greatest hindrance.

—Plato

The all-encompassing nature of HCV treatment can make you feel as if there is nothing else in life. If this is your experience, perhaps you are thinking too much about treatment and not enough about everything else. Although it is important to be vigilant about side effects and other health issues, this vigilance can become a hindrance.

> **Tip for Today:** Just for today, focus on things, people, and activities that bring you joy. Even if you feel lousy, play music or watch a video to divert your thoughts to something else. For one day, leave hepatitis C outside of your field of awareness.

THE FINAL NINE WEEKS

Countdown: 63 days left

And could you keep your heart in wonder at the daily miracles of your life, your pain would not seem less wondrous than your joy.

—Kahlil Gibran

Although the amount of treatment you've completed exceeds that which is ahead of you, the finish line may seem out of sight. Keep doing those practices that sustain you. If side effects are particularly challenging, remember that all you have to do is make it through today, this hour, and this moment.

> **Tip for Today:** Look for the daily miracles in your life. If you can't name any, call a friend, watch something funny on TV, ask for a hug, or find something to lift your spirits. If your mood is low or agitated, be sure to alert your medical provider. It is not too late to try, or adjust the dose of, antidepressant or anti-anxiety medication.

Countdown: 62 days left

When we resist change, it's called suffering. But when we can completely let go and not struggle against it, when we can embrace the groundlessness of our situation and relax into it's dynamic quality, that's called enlightenment.

—Pema Chödrön

Although the side effects of HCV medications are real, resistance can make matters worse. If you resist the reality of what you are coping with, resistance can create its own set of problems or intensify the ones you have. Are you resisting anything?

> **Tip for Today:** For some, headaches are a reality of HCV treatment, a malady made worse by resistance. Headache relief is often a three-step process. First, find the cause, second apply the remedy, and third, don't make the headache worse by resisting the pain. If you have a sinus headache, try steam inhalation, nasal lavage (irrigation), or self-massage to open the sinuses. Hot compresses applied to the sinuses may provide relief. If the headache is caused by tension or muscle spasms, apply cold or hot compresses to the area that hurts most.

Countdown: 61 days left

Dissatisfaction is a great starting point, for it is right there that we have the most power, strength, and energy to push change through.

—David DeNotaris

Your body and your needs may be changing as you go through HCV treatment. This is a good time to check in with yourself, find out what you need, review your goals and recommit to them. You may have new goals to add to your list, such as, *"I want to get through treatment without acting as if I am deranged."*

> **Tip for Today:** Taking care of yourself can come in a variety of forms. You may feel nurtured by nature, church, sporting events or spending time alone or with friends. Perhaps you like to window shop, watch TV, or listen to music. Identify what feeds your spirit and make sure you find ways to meet your needs on a regular basis.

Countdown: 60 days left

Human beings, by changing the inner attitudes of their minds, can change the outer aspects of their lives.

—William James

Thoughts are one of the most influential elements in our lives, and our thoughts can shape our health. Have you ever had an abnormal lab test or lump and worked yourself up into a dire state of worry and illness? After your doctor confirmed that there was nothing serious, did you notice that you felt better? That is the power of the mind to influence health.

> **Tip for Today:** We tell our kids to think big, believe in themselves, and understand that they can do anything they want to. At some point, we seem to forget that this advice applies to us, too. A positive mental attitude may be applied to anything, including HCV treatment. What are you saying to yourself about treatment? Is it an ordeal or an opportunity? You get to decide.

Countdown: 59 days left

Stress is the trash of modern life—we all generate it, but if you don't dispose of it properly, it will pile up and overtake your life.

—Attributed to Danzae Pace

Stress is any physical, chemical, or emotional factor that places tension on the body, mind, or spirit. This tension may disrupt the balance of health and the body's ability to maintain wellness, something that may be in short supply right now. Even mild stress may have long-term harmful effects if it is a constant companion. Imagine holding a one-pound rock at arm's length. Then imagine holding the same rock at arm's length for days or weeks. It would be very painful and damaging. This is much like the effects of chronic stress, so even if you just have a little stress in your life, it is best to manage it now.

> **Tip for Today:** Evaluate your stress level. Are you feeling overwhelmed? Is life out of control, even just a little? A common indicator of stress is that small things bother you more easily. If stress is a problem, implement some stress reduction techniques, such as meditation or pursuing pleasurable activities. Stress reduction is good for your health, and life will be more enjoyable.

Countdown: 58 days left

There are many things to be grateful "for" but, as I ripen with the seasons of life, the many reasons blend into a sacred mystery. And, most deeply, I realize that living gratefully is its own blessing.
—Michael Mahoney

Gratitude is both a state of grace and a way to create one. The opposite, the feeling that everything is wrong, is a form of hell. However, sometimes a feeling of gratitude comes in the midst of the worst circumstances. The trick is to look for it, to call up gratitude when you least feel it, and be willing to practice it under all circumstances.

> **Tip for Today:** As you go to sleep, use your fingers to count 10 things for which you are grateful. Upon awakening, greet the day with a thank you. By framing the day with gratitude, we claim a peace that is beyond what side effects do to us. Practice gratitude throughout the day, especially when your mood is low or resentments creep in.

Countdown: 57 days left

The unendurable is the beginning of the curve of joy.
—Djuna Barnes

At first glance, today's quote may seem outlandish. At your lowest, joy may be the furthest feeling from your mind. But stop and think about this for a moment—treatment does not go on forever. You will get to the end, and from there you will get your life back.

> **Tip for Today:** You are headed into the home stretch, but you still have some distance to travel. Quitting may seem unimaginable at this point, but now is not a good time to get complacent about your treatment. Joy is just around the curve.

FINAL EIGHT WEEKS

Countdown: 56 days left

Just when the caterpillar thought the world was over, it became a butterfly.

—*Origin unknown*

As you near the finish line, you may be tempted to quit. With only eight weeks left, your brain may say, "What if I stop now? How bad would that be?" This is your dear, weary self, longing for a sweet reprieve. Don't be mad at your subconscious, but don't give in to it either.

> **Tip for Today:** Think about something you want to do when treatment is over. Promise yourself that when you are feeling better you will do something you really relish. You won't feel good right away, but you will eventually, and when you do, it will be heavenly. It will be better than being a butterfly.

Countdown: 55 days left

Order is not pressure which is imposed on society from without, but an equilibrium which is set up from within.

—*José Ortega y Gasset*

There is order in your life. You may not feel it, and it may only be apparent to your liver, but a deep organized healing is occurring in your cells. It may take a leap of faith to believe this, but here is the truth: you have everything you need inside of you. Sometimes it may be hard to claim this inner wisdom, but it is there.

Tip for Today: This qigong exercise is purported to help with fatigue. Stand in the position discussed on Day 93 or sit in the position presented on Day 178. Hold your hands about six inches apart, slightly cupped. Imagine you are holding a warm, glowing ball of energy that is growing between your palms. Roll it, stretch it, and play with it, letting it grow as large as you can. Do this for three to five minutes. When you are done, rub your hands together vigorously; and shake them as if you are shaking off water. Let your arms return to their starting position and end with an inhalation and exhalation.

Countdown: 54 days left

Water is the driving force of all nature.
—Leonardo da Vinci

You may be getting tired of water, but remember that hydration is one of the most effective tools to help battle side effects. Assess your fluid intake, and if you aren't drinking enough, try to boost this.

Tip for Today: To increase water intake, find ways to make drinking more enjoyable. Fill a pitcher or glass jar with water and add fresh produce, such as berries, cucumbers, apples, or citrus. Try a water enhancer, such as MiO liquid, a sucralose-based drink mix which comes in multiple flavors. Note: If you use MiO Energy, don't drink it late in the day as it has caffeine.

Countdown: 53 days left

Prayer is not asking. It is a longing of the soul. It is a daily admission of one's weakness.
—Gandhi

During HCV treatment, it sometimes feels as if the internal chatter is tuned to one channel—a negative one. What if I never feel better after hepatitis C treatment? What if my brain always stays foggy? What if I can't make it to the end of treatment? These are words of the mind, but not of the heart. These thoughts constrict and press, keeping the thinker focused on the problem rather than on the present. The present holds the key to peace. Listening to fear is not the path to truth. The way out is to listen to the heart. The heart does not lie.

Tip for Today: Spend a quiet moment listening to your heart. If it feels hard to tune into your deepest wisdom, try listening to the sounds around you. Notice the songs of birds, the rain on a window, or your favorite music. Let the sun warm your face, the snow cool your hands. Read inspiring words, call a friend. Let your heart lead you to health.

Countdown: 52 days left

Dance, even if you have nowhere to do it but your living room.
—*Kurt Vonnegut*

Hepatitis C treatment can make us not want to dance anymore; yet dancing is precisely the thing we need most. Dancing is a metaphor for vitality. When we are dancing with life, we are engaged and fully alive. Someone said, "You can dance anywhere, even if only in your heart."

Tip for Today: Where do you find pleasure in your life? Are you engaged in activities that bring you joy and peace? Are you able to turn off your worries and ignite passion and joy? If not, what stops you? Imagine one small activity that brings you pleasure, and commit to doing it today.

Countdown: 51 days left

Complaining is silly. Either act or forget.
—*Stefan Sagmeister*

Sometimes we just want to complain, particularly if we have suffered an injustice. We shake our fists at the world, looking for a sympathetic listener who will tell us our concerns are justified. Unfortunately, this just stirs the pot of discomfort. HCV treatment is almost over—this is a good time to cook up something new and fresh rather than to let these negative things simmer.

Tip for Today: What do you feel like complaining about? Is there anything that bothers you that can be fixed or simply let go of? If you feel like holding on to a grievance, consider putting it aside until treatment is over. You can write down your complaint, put it in an envelope, and open it up a month after you are finished taking your HCV drugs.

Countdown: 50 days left

Be willing to be a beginner every single morning.
—Meister Eckhart

With only 50 days left to go, you may feel like you know everything about hepatitis C treatment. Even though you are a seasoned warrior, new ideas and information about how to manage HCV treatment side effects are continually being discovered. If you are willing to be a beginner and learn more, it may help make the last 50 days go more smoothly.

Tip for Today: Spend some time reading about HCV side effect management. Refresh your memory by looking for tips in the index of this book. Read the free side effect management fact sheets and guides at the HCV Advocate website (www .hcvadvocate.org).

THE FINAL SEVEN WEEKS

Countdown: 49 days left

It's not the load that breaks you down—it's the way you carry it.
—Lou Holtz (also attributed to Lena Horne)

Consider yourself rare and lucky if you are not feeling weary of HCV treatment. Although the end is in sight, you may have days when you can't see that end. If this happens, get support, set priorities, and continue to stay as healthy as possible, despite the circumstances.

Tip for Today: Assess the quality of the following, and take appropriate action if you identify an area that is out of balance:
- Do you have any side effects that your medical provider needs to help you with?
- Are you getting enough sleep?
- Are you eating enough and nutritiously?
- Are you engaging in some form of physical activity, such as yoga, short walks, stretching, gardening, and so on?
- Are stress or your emotions causing problems for you?
- Are you isolated?
- Do you include activities in your life that bring you pleasure and make you smile?

Countdown: 48 days left

I take a breath when I have to.

—*Ethel Merman*

Are you breathing? With less than eight weeks to go, you may feel inclined to just grit your teeth and suffer your way to the bitter end. However, you don't have to muscle your way to the finish line—try letting go. Simple breathing exercises can help clear your head and give you a little more energy to help you through.

> **Tip for Today:** Some of the most relaxed people in the world are those who practice some form of meditation or mindfulness. Meditation does not need to be complicated or time-consuming. If you can take a few minutes at various intervals in your day and simply pay attention to your breathing, you will do your body, mind, and spirit some good. If this seems monumentally difficult, try the 3 × 3 method. Mindfully, perform three inhalations and exhalations three times a day. That's all you have to do to get started. If you want, you can extend it to ten inhalations three times a day.

Countdown: 47 days left

If you're afraid of butter, use cream.

—*Julia Child*

You can take today's quote figuratively or literally, unless it's against medical advice. Embrace the spirit of the message by trying new foods or jazzing up old favorites to make them more appealing. Let your imagination run wild. If you are short on imagination, ask some friends to suggest their favorite foods.

> **Tip for Today:** At this point, the goal is to fuel your body and make it to the finish line; this means eating even when you don't feel like it. Your sense of taste may have changed, so tempt your taste buds by trying new ingredients or recipes. Add some broccoli and chives to your mac and cheese; try roasted peppers on your grilled cheese. Nibble on brie with pears; sprinkle cinnamon on your baked sweet potato. Put diced apple and walnuts in your chicken salad, a dash of curry in deviled eggs, or make a fruit salad with oranges, dates, and shredded coconut. If you are running out of ideas of what to try, look through magazines and cookbooks for food ideas. If you are not in the mood to cook, you can vary your diet by ordering a new ethnic food for delivery or take-out.

Countdown: 46 days left

Don't take life seriously because you can't come out of it alive.
—Warren Miller

If you are feeling lifeless, check your pulse. If it's beating, then you have enough life inside to get through to the end. A good dose of humor will help you reach the finish line.

> **Tip for Today:** It may be getting harder to find things to laugh about. Try the Norman Cousins laughter plan. Rent, borrow, and watch some comedies. Saturate life with humor.

Countdown: 45 days left

The first wealth is health.
—Ralph Waldo Emerson

Staying physically active is one of the most valuable tools you can use to help you make it through treatment. Moving your body will help with aches and pains, fatigue, sleep, and depression. Even if you don't feel like getting out of your chair or bed, try moving a little bit every hour.

> **Tip for Today:** There are exercises for every physical condition and limitation. You can exercise in a bed, on a couch, in a chair, or on an airplane. YouTube has a vast collection of fitness videos—everything from couch exercises to Chi Walking. Spark up your day with a new exercise routine.

Countdown: 44 days left

We cannot change anything until we accept it. Condemnation does not liberate, it oppresses.
—C.G. Jung

I have seen hepatitis C patients who go through treatment as if it is a shark eating them alive, and they are trying to escape. Others live with treatment as if it is a winter coat, something they need to wear but will discard when the weather warms up. The difference between these two approaches is acceptance. Acceptance liberates our energy, allowing it to be directed toward healing. When we fight treatment, our energy is spent in the battle. If we accept treatment, our energy is conserved for healing.

> **Tip for Today:** Are you condemning hepatitis C treatment or accepting it? If you are fighting it, can you call a truce, at least for today?

Countdown: 43 days left

And yet, when I look up to the sky, I somehow feel that everything will change for the better, that this cruelty too shall end, that peace and tranquility will return once more.

—Anne Frank

It is uncomfortable to think about this reading, knowing how Anne Frank's life ended. However, Anne's words have helped many through difficulties because she held on to hope through the vilest of circumstances. Her words inspire us when we are at our lowest. When times are tough, look up to the sky and know that serenity will return once more.

> **Tip for Today:** Do those things that bring you peace and tranquility. If you can't think of anything that fits the bill, call a friend and ask for help identifying those things that help keep you centered.

THE FINAL SIX WEEKS

Countdown: 42 days left

Difficulties increase the nearer we approach the goal.

—Johann Wolfgang von Goethe

As you get closer to the end of treatment, you may have days when you feel as if you are pushing a boulder up a hill. Whether you are actually having more difficulties, or are losing stamina, it doesn't really matter. At this point, focus on your goals, do whatever it takes to meet them safely, and enlist support to help you.

Tip for Today: Your goal may be to complete treatment. However, your safety is the top priority. If you have any side effects that you feel are serious, be sure you report these to your medical provider. Resist the temptation to put up with problems—you still have six weeks to go—not long, but too long to suffer.

Countdown: 41 days left

We are always getting ready to live but never living.
—*Ralph Waldo Emerson*

How often we think, "I'll do that later. After I retire, I will do such and such. When I feel better, when I get rid of hepatitis C, when I this or that, then I will..." In short, we postpone really living, forgetting that this precious moment and life are slipping through our hands. Don't watch life go by—live it. Let it consume every inch of you—even if you don't feel up to it.

Tip for Today: It may be realistic to postpone some things until after treatment is over, but that doesn't mean you can't dream about them now. Spend time today dreaming. What are your dreams? What do you want to do, but hear yourself saying "no" or "yes but" to? What stops you from really living? Starting today, imagine that nothing stands between you and happiness.

Countdown: 40 days left

Patience is the art of hoping.
—*Marquis de Vauvenargues*

Do you recall your first 40 days, that legendary benchmark of endurance? Since then, you have endured other spans of 40, especially if your treatment plan is for 48 weeks. Now you are looking at the last 40-day cycle, and the end of treatment is in sight. Patience and hope, which carried you this far, will continue to serve you the last 40 days.

Tip for Today: Take a moment to appreciate the distance you have travelled. The experience of having endured this much will provide you with what you need to make it the rest of the way. Hold fast to this truth: nothing can take patience and hope from you; the fact that you have made it this far demonstrates that you have the necessary qualities to prevail over anything.

Countdown: 39 days left

A good laugh and a long sleep are the two best cures in the doctor's book.
—Irish Proverb

With fewer than 40 days of treatment to go, you may be finding it difficult to laugh, but mirth may help more than anything right now. In India, a man named Madan Kataria started laughter yoga, believing that laughter improves our health. You can trick yourself into laughing by watching others who are engaged in hilarity.

Tip for Today: Don't wait for laughter to come to you—pursue it. Watch amusing videos on the Internet. Check out John Cleese's contagious laughter yoga presentation on YouTube.

Countdown: 38 days left

Expectations are resentments under construction.
—Expression commonly heard at Alcoholics
Anonymous and other 12-step meetings

Most of us have expectations, particularly regarding health care. We expect to receive return calls from our doctor's office and to have appointments be on time. We expect to have plenty of time to talk to our medical provider and to have our lab results sent to our doctor's office. However, these things often don't happen. Health care is overburdened, and those who work in this field are stressed. The current system is inefficient, and mistakes happen.

Accepting this new reality without adding harmful stress to the situation allows us to maintain inner peace. A calm interior illuminates the path to solutions.

> **Tip for Today:** Is anything bothering you? If so, are you contributing to this by your own expectations? Spend a moment examining your expectations, and see if there is a way to let any of these go. Lower expectations are more likely to be realized; no expectations have an even higher yield rate. You can always raise your expectations after treatment is over, although keeping them low is a good life practice.

Countdown: 37 days left

He who takes medicine and neglects to diet wastes the skill of his doctors.
—Chinese Proverb

You are going through HCV treatment to reach a goal. Presumably, it is to eradicate this virus, improve your health, and to improve the quality, possibly the longevity of your life. However, there is more to health than just eliminating HCV. Health is a total package deal that includes taking care of your heart, brain, emotions, teeth, joints, and so on. When you take your HCV drugs, you are helping yourself, but perhaps you can do just a little more to help yourself today.

> **Tip for Today:** Is there something you can do to boost your health today? Have you eaten any fruit or vegetables? Have you gone for a walk? Did you floss your teeth? In addition to assessing your present circumstances, think about what sorts of changes you might want to make when you are done with treatment.

Countdown: 36 days left

How poor are they who have not patience! What wound did ever heal but by degrees?
—William Shakespeare

You may be feeling weary and battered, but as you head into the last five weeks of treatment, your job is to keep body, mind, and spirit strong so you can prevail. Patience and HCV medications are healing your liver, cell by cell.

> **Tip for Today:** When patience runs thin, try distraction. Perhaps you are growing tired of TV, so try audio books and YouTube. Ted.com has interesting videos; search for the funniest or most inspiring.

THE FINAL FIVE WEEKS

Countdown: 35 days left

A boy can learn a lot from a dog: obedience, loyalty, and the importance of turning around three times before lying down.
—Robert Benchley

If you have ever watched dogs or cats, you know they do a lot of stretching. In fact, many animals stretch. Humans can be running around all day and then flop into a chair for the evening. The only stretching they do is reaching for the remote. It's ideal to stretch at regular intervals.

Tip for Today: Stretching and relaxation exercises provide relief for headaches, muscle aches, and other sore areas. Stretch gently while listening to soothing music. After stretching, lie down, breathe deeply, and imagine you are inhaling oxygen right to the sorest spot. When you exhale, imagine the breath carrying the pain out of your body. When you are done, stretch some more before resuming normal activities.

Countdown: 34 days left

I believe that water is the only drink for a wise man.
—Henry David Thoreau

Even though we know that alcohol and hepatitis C are not compatible, it might be tempting to drink during this hard time. Don't do it. Alcohol use is particularly ill-advised during HCV treatment. You have come this far, and staying alcohol-free is an important part of ensuring your continued success. Maintain your resolve to abstain from alcohol until your medical provider advises otherwise.

Tip for Today: If you feel like drinking, mix a special nonalcoholic beverage. Distract yourself with something entertaining. If pain is the reason you want to drink, talk to your medical provider about how to manage this.

Countdown: 33 days left

The best and safest thing is to keep a balance in your life, acknowledge the great powers around us and in us. If you can do that, and live that way, you are really a wise man.

—*Euripides*

If your inner resources feel depleted, look outside and inside of yourself to see what you need to replenish. There are healers all around you, ready to help you determine your needs that will enable you to complete the last month of hepatitis C treatment.

Tip for Today: This qigong exercise is purported to harmonize the liver and spleen. Stand in the position discussed on Day 93 or sit in the position presented on Day 178. Bring hands together in front of your navel and imagine you are holding a small ball of energy. Slowly separate your hands, with one palm facing up, the other facing down. Breathe and imagine energy moving along your liver and spleen as you move your arms apart. Return the ball to the original position. Turn palms the other way and repeat. Do five to eight times, ending by placing your hands on your liver and spleen, inhaling and exhaling.

Countdown: 32 days left

Hope begins in the dark, the stubborn hope that if you just show up and try to do the right thing, the dawn will come. You wait and watch and work: You don't give up.

—*Anne Lamott*

Although the end of treatment is near, it may feel farther away than when you began. Your body, mind, and spirit may be shouting, "I can't do this anymore!" Still, you do because if you were someone who quit when the going got tough, you would have quit long ago.

Tip for Today: Wait, watch, and don't give up. How do you do this? The same way you have been doing all along, however this works for you. Call a friend, distract yourself, take a nap, go for a walk. Need to try something new? Look back through some of the tips, and try something you haven't tried before.

Countdown: 31 days left

The making of friends who are real friends, is the best token we have of a man's success in life.

—*Edward Everett Hale*

In 2009, Tara Parker-Pope of *The New York Times* reported on a study at the University of Virginia that outfitted each of 34 enrolled students with heavy backpacks. They were taken to the base of a hill and asked to estimate its steepness. Some participants stood next to friends, while others were alone during the exercise. Those who stood with friends gave lower estimates of the hill's steepness. The longer the friendship, the less steep the hill appeared.

Tip for Today: Talk to a friend who you have known for a long time and spend quality time walking up the last steep part of treatment. You don't have to do much; just be together.

Countdown: 30 days left

Learn to say "no." It will be of more use to you than to be able to read Latin.

—*Charles H. Spurgeon*

Forty days may be the legendary biblical mark of time for major accomplishments, but 30 days also has symbolic qualities. Thirty days is the average calendar month. Thirty days is all that is left to this treatment. Surely, you can make it with less than a month left.

Tip for Today: *To help make it to the finish line, keep your obligations to a minimum. Say "no" to anything you don't want to do or to things that can wait until you have completed HCV therapy. If it can't wait, delegate it. The word "no" is a complete sentence; use it freely.*

Countdown: 29 days left

Warning: Humor may be hazardous to your illness.

—*Ellie Katz*

Today's quote is a reminder to include humor in your life. You have worked so hard to get this far that you are probably needing a good laugh.

Tip for Today: With the finish line so close, it may be tempting to grit your teeth and just get through treatment. However, now is not the time to skimp on self-care. Find ways to laugh and lighten your load.

THE FINAL FOUR WEEKS

Countdown: 28 days left

Don't take your organs to heaven—heaven knows we need them here.
—Bosco's Buddies website

People with HCV may not donate blood, but they can be organ donors. Patients with HCV who are waiting for life-saving organs are sometimes given the option of accepting healthy organs that test positive for HCV. With the critical organ shortage, choosing a healthy HCV-positive organ may mean the difference between life and death.

Tip for Today: Being a potential organ donor is an easy way to do something for someone else, even if you aren't helping someone at that precise moment. Registering as an organ donation is easy. For information, visit the DonateLife website.

Countdown: 27 days left

What would life be if we had no courage to attempt anything?
—Vincent van Gogh

If you had not attempted treatment, your liver would still be under constant attack. HCV replicates a trillion times every day. The liver fights back, launching a cascade of chemical responses, but in the end, people with HCV live with constant inflammation and liver damage. When taking antiviral medications, the liver gets a reprieve from HCV's relentless assault.

Tip for Today: Spend a moment appreciating your courage—not just the bravery it took to start HCV treatment, but the daily strength it takes to face the challenges of this treatment. You could have quit taking the medications, but you didn't. Courage will carry you through this last month of treatment.

Countdown: 26 days left

If you can spend a perfectly useless afternoon in a perfectly useless manner, you have learned how to live.

—Lin Yutang

Setting lofty goals and staying positive are wonderful ideals, but when one is fatigued, it can feel impossible to meet these objectives. Sometimes the best way to deal with bone-tired exhaustion is to just lie down and let time pass.

Tip for Today: When tired, you may feel as if you will never get your life back. Don't let negative thoughts intrude—these thoughts are untrue and just make matters worse. You will get your life back eventually.

Countdown: 25 days left

The heart is cooking a pot of food for you. Be patient until it is cooked.

—Rumi

Patience will help you endure the last 25 days of treatment, but without fuel for your body, patience is useless. Focus on quick, easy, filling foods to fortify you so you can make it through these last few weeks.

Tip for Today: If you are running out of ideas of things to eat, e-mail family and friends or post a message to Facebook, requesting suggestions. Try ready-made protein drinks or shakes from the drive-thru of your favorite fast food restaurant. Mashed potatoes with melted cheese provide lots of calories. Frozen yogurt may soothe a dry, aching mouth. Want something really healthy? Get a vegetable and fruit juice from your local health food store.

Countdown: 24 days left

Whenever feeling downcast, each person should vitally remember, "For my sake, the entire world was created."

—Baal Shem Tov

Although you are close to completing HCV treatment, your body and brain are likely feeling downtrodden. You may be trying to "muscle through" the last few weeks of treatment. However, your medical provider may be able to help with medications to treat your moods, sleep issues, or physical complaints.

Tip for Today: If you are feeling low, talk to your medical provider about how to make it through the next few months. Be sure you are evaluated for thyroid abnormalities and other medical conditions that cause depression or anxiety. Keep in mind that although you are almost done with treatment, it may be weeks or months before your mental health stabilizes. Don't rule out the potential help that medications can bring. Even if you only take them for a couple of months, it may help you get back on your feet sooner.

Countdown: 23 days left

Our entire life...consists ultimately in accepting ourselves as we are.
—Jean Anouilh

It isn't always easy to accept that we are who we are and even harder to accept others as they are. If you are in a relationship, your sex life may have stopped. A romantic evening may constitute watching TV with you snoring on the couch. Life will get better, particularly if both you and your partner are patient and kind with each other.

Tip for Today: Thank your partner for all he or she has endured so far. Reassure your partner that life will get better, not immediately after you are done taking antiviral mediations, but in time. Try holding hands and appreciate what your partner is also giving up in order to gain a better life with you.

Countdown: 22 days left

The best things in life are nearest: Breath in your nostrils, light in your eyes, flowers at your feet, duties at your hand, the path of right just before you. Then do not grasp at the stars, but do life's plain, common work as it comes, certain that daily duties and daily bread are the sweetest things in life.
—Robert Louis Stevenson

As you round the corner of treatment, this is a perfect moment to look at how short the path is in front of you compared to the length you have travelled. You walked this path not only breath by breath and heartbeat by heartbeat, but pill by pill and side effect by side effect.

Tip for Today: Take a moment to savor the ordinary pleasures in life—a piece of bread with butter, the front steps swept of leaves, a cup of hot tea, the morning sun, or a gentle rain ushering in the day.

THE FINAL THREE WEEKS

Countdown: 21 days left

Everything done in the world is done by hope.

—Martin Luther

Hope helped you take the first step and supported you through HCV treatment. Although you are almost done, you still need hope. Hang on to optimism, even if it is only a thin thread. If you lose hope, start looking for it. You will find it on children's faces, in nature, among those who attend HCV groups, and in the hearts of anyone who ever scaled the steep cliffs of life.

Tip for Today: You need hope, but you also need adequate hydration. You may be getting sick of drinking fluids, but sufficient water intake is critical. If you have reached the point where you cannot stomach the thought of another glass of water, try flavored waters and teas. You can buy them already mixed or make your own. Mix lemonade or fruit juice with club soda. Drink tonic water, club soda, or fruit juice. Be careful of sugar, and brush your teeth so you don't end up with a cavity at the end of treatment.

Countdown: 20 days left

We should look for someone to eat and drink with before looking for something to eat and drink.

—Epicurus

The end of treatment is close. At this point, your biggest challenge may be to just to hang on. Remember to eat, find ways to laugh, and avoid isolation.

> **Tip for Today:** Why wait until you are done with treatment to celebrate? The end will be cause enough to feel good. There is no reason why you can't honor the fact that you are almost finished with HCV treatment. Ask a friend to host a potluck for you to which guests bring their favorite comfort foods. If you host this, don't clean in advance, and ask someone to stay and tidy up afterward.

Countdown: 19 days left

Take a music bath once or twice a week for a few seasons, and you will find that it is to the soul what the water bath is to the body.
—*Oliver Wendell Holmes*

Pleasure is essential in life, and during HCV treatment, it may be hard to find activities that bring much enjoyment. Even a little delight is better than none at all. Pleasure helps the immune system, cardiovascular system, and is good for your overall health. It also makes the time easier to endure.

> **Tip for Today:** Bathe yourself in anything that feels good—assuming it is healthy. Take a hot bath in mineral salts, listen to your favorite music, watch a sporting event on TV, or surf the web for your favorite sites.

Countdown: 18 days left

Take more time, cover less ground.
—*Thomas Merton*

The finish line is in view. Staying in the present will help your battered body through the last part of treatment. Mindfulness helps you maintain balance so when you walk, you reduce the risk of falling or bumping into things. By focusing only on the task at hand, you decrease your accident risk.

> **Tip for Today:** Drive while driving. Walk while walking. Cook while cooking. Keep distractions to a minimum by turning off the TV, radio, phone, and other unnecessary intrusions. Try to make it to the end of treatment without stubbing your toe, denting a fender, or something worse.

Countdown: 17 days left

A friend is someone who knows the song in your heart, and can sing it back to you when you have forgotten the words.

—Unknown

Family and friends want to support their loved ones during HCV treatment, even though they may not know how. The problem is that it can be difficult for patients to identify what they need. They want to be supported but don't have a clue as to what they need. In an ideal world, everyone would have someone who knows them so well that they can feel supported even when they don't know what they need.

> **Tip for Today:** Is there someone in your life who knows you really well, someone who has a knack for saying the right thing when you need it most? Perhaps you have a friend you aren't in constant contact with but who usually makes you feel better when you talk to him or her. If no one fits that description, perhaps there is someone you can call and say, "I need someone to listen to me who won't try to fix my problems."

Countdown: 16 days left

Those who dream by day are cognizant of many things which escape those who dream only by night.

—Edgar Allan Poe

Daydreaming is one of the loveliest escapes. With nothing more than your imagination, you can dream of going to a secluded beach or the Olympics or anything your heart desires. Imagination is a good use of time, especially if it leads us to follow our dreams.

> **Tip for Today:** Spend time daydreaming about what you want after treatment is over. What do you want to eat? Where do you want to go? What do you want to do? Who do you want to see? Imagine a life free from hepatitis C.

Countdown: 15 days left

Difficult times have helped me to understand better than before, how infinitely rich and beautiful life is in every way, and that so many things that one goes worrying about are of no importance whatsoever.

—Isak Dinesen

One of the gifts of HCV treatment is perspective, bestowed because of the difficult nature of this regimen. The daily grueling grind is awful, but later, most patients look back at this time and realize what is important and what isn't. They also see how strong they are and use that strength to help them endure future challenges.

> **Tip for Today:** Take a moment to reflect on anything that may be bothering you. Are you fretting over important issues or ones that really aren't important in the grand scheme of life? Although worrying is not a good use of one's time, at the very least, try to limit your worrying to priority problems that are solvable. Clearing the head of distressful thoughts makes room for calm ones.

THE FINAL TWO WEEKS

Countdown: 14 days left

Patience and time do more than strength or passion.
—Jean de La Fontaine

Patience is strength. At this point, you probably feel at an all-time low, physically as well as emotionally. However, feelings don't describe the truth, which is that you are strong even if you don't feel it. The proof lies in the fact that you have made this journey despite relentless side effects. Anyone can muster up patience if they feel good, but the strong ones are those who plod along when feeling weak.

> **Tip for Today:** After today's injection, you only have one more shot. Let this fact sink in, relish it, and know that better days are ahead.

Countdown: 13 days left

One good thing about music, when it hits you, you feel no pain.
—Bob Marley

With less than two weeks to go, distraction may be the most reliable tool for enduring side effects. Find ways to keep your mind off your problems, and you can endure just about anything.

Tip for Today: Here are some ideas to help distract you from discomfort: Music, TV, the movies (with popcorn), audio books, YouTube, solitaire, computer games, time with friends, a museum, sporting events, sleeping, being in nature.

Countdown: 12 days left

The crisis of today is the joke of tomorrow.

—*H.G. Wells*

In the midst of agony when people say, "Someday you will look back on this and laugh," my reaction is, "Why not laugh at it today?" You are very close to the end of treatment; why not make the best of every minute? You will not miss using your skin as a pin cushion or having a perpetually cloudy brain, but at least laugh at the experience. It beats crying.

Tip for Today: Squeeze a smile out of some aspect of treatment. If you can't find anything to laugh at, hang in there; your humor will return.

Countdown: 11 days left

An optimist isn't necessarily a blithe, sappy whistler in the dark. To be hopeful in bad times is not just foolishly romantic. If we remember those times and places where people have behaved magnificently, this gives us energy to act and at least the possibility of sending this spinning top of a world in a different direction.

—*Howard Zinn*

You may be wondering about the outcome of treatment, whether you will have a permanent response. Try to remain optimistic. Statistics are on your side, and the fact that you have made it this far in treatment gives you even more reason to remain optimistic.

Tip for Today: Getting sidetracked by "what ifs" is not a good use of your brain. If you are caught up in speculation, remind yourself that your liver is benefiting from treatment. You have already succeeded.

Countdown: 10 days left

What brings fulfillment is gratefulness, the simple response of our heart to this life in all its fullness.

—*David Steindl-Rast*

Gratitude is an art, a gift, and a practice best performed when we are feeling the least grateful. The paradox is that gratitude is most powerful when we feel we have little to appreciate. By making a conscious decision to appreciate the gifts in life, we can find pleasure and hope in simple things, especially when things seem rough. The feeling of gratitude for an orange, a bowl of rice, or the glow of a full moon can lift the most troubled heart.

Tip for Today: Reflect back on your treatment and make a list of things for which you are grateful. If you can't think of anything, here is one to get you started: I am grateful that I have made it through treatment and only have one more shot to go.

Countdown: 9 days left

Success is sweet and sweeter if long delayed and gotten through many struggles and defeats.

—*Amos Bronson Alcott*

Success certainly has been long-delayed, and soon you will be walking out of this turbulent experience. As you round the corner on treatment, know that success is in the effort, not the outcome. You have already succeeded in making it this far.

Tip for Today: You have nearly achieved your goals, and at this point, nothing but time stands between you and the finish line. After you begin to feel better, what do you want to do to begin enjoying your life again? Spend a little time daydreaming about possibilities.

Countdown: 8 days left

For the person who has learned to let go and let be, nothing can ever get in the way again.

—*Meister Eckhart*

One of the unexpected benefits of HCV treatment is something that you may not yet have recognized in yourself, but will in the future, and that is the gift of confidence. HCV treatment is a monumental trial of endurance, and later on, when looking back at what you have accomplished, you may feel as if there is nothing you can't achieve in the future.

> **Tip for Today:** You are almost finished with treatment. At the end of today when you take your pills, say to yourself, "Tomorrow marks my last week, and my last shot. I achieved so much."

THE FINAL WEEK

Note: The final week of readings assumes that you are on the last stretch of treatment. Although extended treatment is rare, this decision may be made late in the game. If your medical provider has extended your treatment, postpone this week's readings until the last week of treatment. Stop here, and fill in with extra daily readings found in any portion of this book that you found particularly helpful. Expanded treatment can be discouraging news; try your best to stay positive and focused on taking care of yourself.

Countdown: 7 days left

Fear cannot be without hope nor hope without fear.
—Benedict de Spinoza

You made it to your last injection and your last week. Fantastic! You may be wondering if your efforts have paid off. This is a time for hope. Anxiety and fear are frequent companions of true hope, so don't be dismayed if these feelings come up. Hang your hat on hope, and the fear will slip away.

> **Tip for Today:** Celebrate your last injection. On one of the Facebook HCV groups, patients invite members to have "last shot" virtual parties. Another way to mark the occasion is disposing of your needles and syringes. Assuming you stored them in a "sharps" container, return used needles and syringes to your pharmacist or medical provider. Some communities have drop-off points for needles, syringes, and unused medications. Not only are you done with injections, you are regaining a needle-free space in your life.

Countdown: 6 days left

Anything I've ever done that ultimately was worthwhile initially scared me to death.

—Betty Bender

If you are like me, you were scared before you started treatment. Now, here you are near the finish line. Courage is action taken in the face of fear. There is no question that you are brave, a fact to remember as you face the days ahead. Although you are almost finished with your HCV medications, you have more work ahead of you.

> **Tip for Today:** The end of treatment, along with the days, weeks, and months following it are fragile and unpredictable. Patients think they will feel better quickly, which is often not the case. Plan to continue applying side effect management techniques, such as drinking plenty of water, engaging in light exercise, getting sufficient rest, taking care of your skin, and so on, until side effects are firmly resolved.

Countdown: 5 days left

A hug a day keeps the demons at bay.

—German Proverb

Now that you are on the home stretch, it can be tempting to reject help from others. After all, the fact that you made it this far shows how strong you are. However, just as a racehorse can't win a race without a jockey, your end of treatment will go more smoothly if you accept help and support from others.

> **Tip for Today:** When was the last time you got a hug or some sort of support? If it has been a while, perhaps you can contact someone who knows how to make you feel good. If you don't want support, reach out and give support to someone else who needs it, perhaps to a person who is starting HCV treatment.

Countdown: 4 days left

Patience: To wait with certainty; the art of allowing life to carry you.

—Chinese Proverb

It is likely that your body, mind, and spirit are anxious to begin the work of feeling better. Your family and friends are probably anxious, too, having watched you disappear into a fog of side effects for many months. However, most people don't just return to their pretreatment state the day the last hepatitis C drug is taken. It takes weeks, months, and sometimes longer before the body feels completely normal.

> **Tip for Today:** Talk to your family, friends, and co-workers about what may be ahead. Ask for their continued support and patience during this transition as you come off HCV medications. Acknowledge that you understand that it has been a hard time for them, too. Yes, it has been much harder for you than for others, but that does not diminish their struggles while witnessing your pain.

Countdown: 3 days left

We must always change, renew, rejuvenate ourselves; otherwise we harden.
—*Johann Wolfgang von Goethe*

An irony of taking hepatitis C medications is that although this time-consuming therapy is healing the liver, the patient needs to heal from the treatment. In two days, you will finish taking your HCV drugs and begin a new phase of healing.

> **Tip for Today:** Resist the temptation to make plans for the first few months after treatment. You don't know how quickly you will bounce back. However, dream all you want about what you will do when you are feeling better.

Countdown: 2 days left

He conquers who endures.

—*Persius*

You conquered because you endured, and you endured because you conquered. You may feel as if you were a slave to HCV medications and their side effects, but you were the master because you made it through treatment.

> **Tip for Today:** At the end of today when you take your pills, say to yourself, "Tomorrow is the last day I will take HCV drugs." The end of treatment is almost here.

The Last Day

No one knows what he can do till he tries.

—*Publilius Syrus*

Congratulations, you did it! You succeeded in completing HCV treatment, something that many are too afraid to even attempt. Self-doubt and questions about your strength and ability to endure the side effects can be put to rest. Completing HCV treatment is the proof of how strong and courageous you are.

Although you have been anticipating this moment, don't be surprised if reaching this milestone feels anticlimactic. You may be feeling too sick and tired to enjoy the accomplishment. If you don't feel like celebrating, then don't. You have the rest of your life to celebrate, a life you have honored by enduring hepatitis C treatment, one step at a time. If you are in a celebratory mood, then by all means, celebrate—you earned it.

Tip for Today: Do something special to mark this milestone. Even if you don't feel like doing much, tell someone about your accomplishment. If you belong to a support group, celebrate your success with the group.

7

●●●●●○

Waiting for Results

Somewhere, something incredible is waiting to be known.

—*Carl Sagan*

Now that you are done with treatment, you may be feeling a mixture of emotions. You may be happy that you are done, but feeling a little lost, like someone who quit their job—happy that it is over but wondering what to do with yourself now. At the same time, you may feel low and infirmed, since your body is still under the influence of medications.

The chief question for most patients is, "When will I feel better?" Recovery times vary, but don't count on bouncing back immediately. It takes time, and progress rarely occurs in a straight line. Some patients feel better in a month, some in a year; most fall somewhere in the middle. Some patients say that when they did start to feel well, they felt better than they had prior to treatment, particularly patients who sustain a response to treatment.

I have observed that patients often get sick after finishing their HCV medications. My theory is that without extra interferon to ward off viruses and bacteria, we are now just as susceptible as everyone else is to common "bugs." Plus, now we are getting out more and may be exposed to more microorganisms. Although illness does seem to occur frequently in this posttreatment stage, don't be alarmed. In time, your body's natural immunity will begin protecting you the way it is supposed to.

You may be thinking about the future—wondering if the virus you have lived with so long is permanently gone. You invested a lot to get to this point, and, naturally, you want the best possible outcome. Try to live in the present, and leave the question alone. Worry and speculation just add a layer of discomfort and will not provide you with an answer any sooner. Besides, there is a more pressing need at hand—the business of reclaiming your health.

Here are some key issues for the posttreatment recovery period:

- Women who could become pregnant must continue to avoid pregnancy for six months after finishing HCV treatment. Female partners of men who were treated must also avoid pregnancy for six months. Continue to use two effective forms of birth control.
- Schedule follow-up lab testing and medical appointments. Your medical provider will advise you how often you need to do this. If medical problems occur between appointments, be sure to report these and be seen accordingly.
- Continue to take medications that were prescribed for HCV treatment side effects and other medical issues, especially antidepressant medication. Abrupt stopping of antidepressant medications can be dangerous. It takes time for your brain to start making the necessary chemicals to help you feel better, and experts recommend a gradual reduction in antidepressant dosage. Sometimes this is delayed for months before beginning this slow process. Your medical provider will discuss the safest way to taper off medications.
- Properly dispose of any unused HCV medication, needles, and syringes. These can usually be taken to your pharmacy or medical provider's office.
- Do not drink alcohol or take any drugs or medications unless medically-sanctioned.
- Avoid risk of future HCV exposure. Although you have the HCV antibody, this does not protect you against reinfection. Just like anyone, you can contract HCV again through contaminated sources, such as shared injection drug use or blood transfusions in foreign countries where the blood supply may be unsafe.
- Continue to take care with your blood. Even if you are cured of HCV, it is best to take the same precautions as health care professionals do—act as if *all* blood may carry something potentially infectious.

As you start to feel better, this is an opportune time to build up your health. Here are some suggestions:

- Increase exercise intensity or start a regular physical fitness program as soon as you can. If you have not done much, start with five minutes. If five minutes is too much, start with one minute. The goal is to build strength, which will help your bones, brain, mood, and sleep, among other health benefits.

- Reclaim your social life. If you have isolated yourself in the past weeks, schedule time with people and pursue activities that lift your mood.
- If your sex life slacked off during treatment, your partner may be missing the intimacy. Mae West said, "Sex is emotion in motion," so when you feel better, reclaim your sex life.
- If you made changes to your work or went on disability, talk to your medical provider about when you may be able to return to work. It is usually best to return gradually rather than all at once.
- Continue to drink six to eight glasses of water every day.
- Include humor in your recovery plan. You may be done with HCV treatment, but you are not done with life; in many ways, you are just beginning. Humor can smooth life's rough spots.

Generally, the final HCV viral load is performed at six months following the end of treatment. A *nondetectable* or *undetectable* result means that you are cured. This is the best possible outcome. Since the chances are less than one-half of a percent that HCV will return, you can assume this means HCV is permanently gone as long as you never expose yourself to it again.

HCV viral load results can be confusing. *Nondetectable* means you are cured, but sometimes the results are written: *less than 15 or < 15 IU/L*. This means that the test used to measure HCV in your blood could not find any HCV. This test is sensitive, and if you had 16 IU/L, it would have shown up. Given that HCV replicates a trillion times a day, you can be sure that you are cured with results like this.

Patients may find it more difficult to be confident when a viral load test uses a higher range, and they receive results that are something like *nondetectable at <600 IU/L*. But, think about this: if HCV replicates a trillion times a day, the chances that you have 599 IU/L just sitting in your blood and not replicating in your liver are close to zero.

Human beings are rarely satisfied with a single test result. I've known patients who asked their medical providers to repeat the test in a year, and some patients have had the test repeated a few more times after that before they finally believed that HCV was truly gone. Discuss this with your medical provider, and figure out for yourself what you need to feel confident that you are permanently free of hepatitis C.

When you start to feel better, you may keep improving for many years. Research shows us that HCV patients who are cured have longer, healthier, better-quality lives. Patients report improved mental clarity, an improvement supported by brain imaging scans. In short, get rid of hepatitis C, get a better life back.

Although you no longer have hepatitis C, you will continue to test positive for the HCV antibody. The antibody cannot hurt you any more than a picture of a snake can. If you apply for life insurance, typically you will be tested for HCV. You can ask your doctor to write a letter saying that although you test positive for HCV, you are cured.

A small portion of you will have the outcome I had—a return of HCV. Patients who experience this are referred to as *responder-relapsers.* I call them heroes, since this small group must courageously go forward without the wings of success to hold them up. The next chapter is for you.

One thing is certain regardless of the outcome—you accomplished a huge feat. The final lab results do not alter the fact that you successfully completed treatment. You will always know that you are capable of enduring incredible hardship, so celebrate this achievement. You earned it.

8

●●●●●○

When Treatment Doesn't Work

Nothing is a waste of time if you use your experience wisely.
—Auguste Rodin

Approximately twenty percent of you who tried HCV treatment will
have reason to read this chapter. You have my sympathy and admira-
tion. Since I fell into this category too, I know some of what you may be
experiencing. In plain English, it sucks.

When I went through treatment, everyone who started at the same
time as me ended up with nondetectable HCV, including two men who
had incredibly low odds of being cured; one because he was an African
American with cirrhosis, and the other was coinfected with HIV. My
first response was to wonder what I did wrong. My mind churned on
that for a while before I was able to let that go.

● If you did not respond to treatment, do not beat yourself up. What
is done is done, and you aren't going to help your liver, your health,
or those around you if you dwell in negativity. Rehashing the past
is like doing a postmortem exam, hoping to get different results.
I created a mantra to redirect my thoughts when they got caught up
on this issue—*no postmortems*.

It helped me to look for the good. This didn't happen in the
beginning, but in time, my list grew, filled with genuine gifts
I received despite not being cured. For instance, I definitely had
improved liver tissue, verified by a biopsy. Also, I was glad that I had

been proactive by trying treatment, rather than choosing the other path of letting HCV continue to engulf my liver.

- When you are ready, look for the positive. However, before you do this, read the next suggestion.

Having a good attitude is great, but sometimes we try to push ourselves to be happy before we are ready. Before you accentuate the positive, you need to feel the negative.

- If you feel pain, discomfort, grief, or other strong feelings about your treatment outcome, lean into the feelings. Let them teach you. Just don't hang out there too long. If you need support, talk to a counselor or medical provider.

From a medical standpoint, your liver enzymes and viral load tests may be substantially higher than before. This is normal.

- Don't panic. High lab results do not mean that your health is deteriorating.

One question you may ask is, "What's next?" There are numerous drugs in clinical testing, so many that it can be overwhelming to stay informed. Your medical provider will tell you how much time you can afford to wait and suggest the next course of action to take.

You may have a hard time imagining going through this again. I certainly felt that way, although I managed to find the strength to do three treatments. Because of amazing research advancements, each treatment is more effective, and often easier and/or shorter. If my third treatment does not work, then I will try it again. Although up to now I haven't succeeded in eliminating HCV from my body, there is one thing I have learned how to do—succeed at treatment.

Since I don't know the outcome of my third treatment, I am assessing the data of HCV drugs advancing in the development process. As this book was headed to the publisher, the FDA gave priority review status to two drugs: Janssen's simeprevir and Gilead's sofosbuvir. If simeprevir is approved, its initial indication will be for genotype 1 patients. It is daily pill, taken with peginterferon and ribavirin.

If sofosbuvir is approved, patients with genotype 1, 4, 5 and 6 who have had no prior HCV treatment, may have the option to take this once-daily pill in combination with peginterferon and ribavirin. Genotype 2 and 3 patients may have a chance at an all-oral HCV treatment, combining sofosbuvir with ribavirin. However, the treatment response rates for genotype 3 patients were significantly lower than genotype 2, so this group may have better odds with peginterferon and ribavirin. Gilead has other HCV drugs in development and will likely have an all-oral treatment soon.

AbbVie is researching an unnamed, multi-drug HCV treatment that is so promising that the FDA has designated it as *breakthrough therapy*. This triggers a fast track feature, and this is the first group of HCV agents to get this designation.

Other pharmaceutical companies that are further along in the drug development process are Boehringer Ingelheim, and Bristol-Myers Squibb. Also, watch Achillion, Genentech, Idenix, Merck, and Vertex. There are others companies researching HCV treatments. Information about these may be found under "Clinical Trials and Research" in the Resources guide.

In the interim, your principal job is to take care of your health. For information on this and other posttreatment issues, the Hepatitis C Support Project offers a free booklet, *Next Steps: When Treatment Isn't Working*, which can be downloaded at www.hcvadvocate.org.

No matter what you decide, may you enjoy your precious life. You gave up a great deal to go through treatment. You don't have to let hepatitis C ruin your future. Treatment is over; your life is ahead of you.

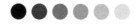

CONCLUSION

Act as if what you do makes a difference. It does.

—*William James*

You have endured and triumphed through an amazing ordeal—hepatitis C treatment. Regardless of the outcome, you can claim victory because you competed. You did not sit on the sidelines and let HCV devour your liver or your future. You fought back.

Rest for a while, build your strength back, and when you are ready, consider this: What can you do to help others? What can you do to help create a world free from hepatitis C?

You may wonder if you have anything to offer, and while considering this, I offer a story about President Kennedy. The story may be true, or it may be an urban legend, but it is still a good story. While touring the NASA facility the president asked a janitor, "What do you do here at NASA?" The janitor replied, "I am helping to put a man on the moon."

I am not asking you to send a person to the moon. I am asking for something even bigger—to help save lives—millions of them. I am inviting you to help erase hepatitis C from the planet. I know you can help because you were strong enough to endure HCV treatment. However, it isn't strength alone that will change the world; it takes teamwork.

How can you help? Tell your story. Urge Congress to support funding for HCV testing, treatment, and research. Raise public awareness by writing to your local newspaper. Use the Internet and social media to educate others. Start an HCV support group. Be a beacon of hope and start climbing to lofty heights, one step at a time.

Appendix A

● ● ● ● ● ●

Foods with 20 Grams of Fat

NOTE: Telaprevir is to be taken with 20 grams of fat. Telaprevir is taken for 12 weeks, and after that, patients can resume a regular diet.

- Avocado—1 cup
- Bacon—2 ounces, cooked
- Butter—1 ounce
- Cheese, hard such as cheddar, jack, Swiss, and so forth—2 to 2.5 ounces
- Cheese, soft such as blue, camembert, goat, and so forth—2.5 to 3 ounces
- Cheese, low-fat semi-hard such as mozzarella, Muenster, and so forth—4 to 5 ounces
- Chocolate, dark—2 ounces
- Coconut, dried—1+ ounces
- Cooking oil (olive is among the healthiest; canola, sunflower, soy, and safflower are other healthy oils)—4 teaspoons
- Cream cheese, full-fat—2 ounces
- Croissants—2 medium
- Eggnog, full fat—1 cup
- Eggs with yolks—4 large
- Flax seed oil—1.5 tablespoons
- Hamburger patty (75% lean/25% fat)—4 ounces

- Ice cream (full-fat, vanilla)—1.5 cups
- Italian salad dressing—5 tablespoons
- Mayonnaise—4 tablespoons
- Milk, whole—2.5 cups
- Milkshake—20 ounces
- Nuts such as almonds, walnuts, pistachios—1/3 cup
- Olives—4 large
- Omelet—2 large eggs, 1 ounce cheese cooked in 1 teaspoon of butter
- Peanut butter, almond butter, and so forth—2.5 tablespoons
- Pizza—2–2.5 slices of a 14" pie
- Ranch salad dressing—2.5 tablespoons
- Roasted chicken with skin—6 to 10 ounces
- Salmon—6 ounces (20 ounces smoked salmon)
- Sardines in oil—3 ounces
- Sour cream—1/2 cup
- Starbucks Café Mocha—Any grande or venti size made with whole milk and whipped cream
- Sunflower seeds—1/3 cup
- Trail mix—1/2 cup
- Tuna salad—3 ounces with 1 tablespoon of mayo
- Yogurt, plain whole milk—20 ounces

Appendix B

●●●●●●

Managing Anal/Rectal Discomfort

- Keep the anal area clean. Gently cleanse with a soft wet cloth, paper towel, unscented wipe, or squeezable water bottle.
- Be sure area is dry. Pat dry with toilet paper or soft paper towel. A hair dryer at a low setting is a good way to dry the area. Cornstarch, talc, or baby powder may keep the area dry.
- Avoid irritants, such as bubble bath, perfumes, or scented soaps. Use unbleached, unscented toilet paper.
- Protect your skin with A & D ointment, Balneol lotion, or a zinc oxide product such as Desitin.
- Many products provide relief for anal/rectal problems. Preparation H offers a variety of ointments; look for one that suits your needs. For mild-to-moderate anal itching, try over-the-counter creams or ointments that contain hydrocortisone. Use these sparingly and as directed.
- If these measures don't work, your medical provider may prescribe a cream or ointment and/or an antihistamine.
- Try not to scratch, as this increases the itch and further irritates the skin. Sitz baths and cold compresses may help relieve itching. A sitz bath is a warm bath that covers the buttocks. A regular tub is suitable.
- Wear natural fiber underwear and loose clothing. Avoid pantyhose and tight-fitting garments.
- If diarrhea or loose stools remain a problem, speak to your medical provider.

ADDITIONAL RESOURCES

www.incivek.com/hcp/anorectal-adverse-events

www.hcvadvocate.org/hepatitis/factsheets_pdf/SEM_Anal%
20Itching.pdf

Appendix C

●●●●●●

Managing Skin Problems

All HCV medications, especially telaprevir and ribavirin, may cause skin problems. Those taking telaprevir need to be aware of the strong warning associated with this medication for serious skin reactions. Although these reactions are rare, they are potentially fatal. Of those taking telaprevir, 6 percent discontinue this medication due to severe rash; 1 percent discontinue all of their HCV treatment because of a rash. See full prescribing information for a complete warning.

Since more than half of patients get some sort of rash, it is critical to learn how to manage skin problems and to know the difference between a mild-to-moderate problem and a severe one. A mild rash is confined to a few small areas of the body, such as on the hands and chest. The rash may or may not itch. A moderate rash is spread over more of the body. The skin may be beginning to peel, and again, it may or may not itch. A severe rash has significant skin breakdown, such as blisters and ulcers. There is often itching, but not always, and a severe rash is usually over much of the body. It can be bright red, like sunburn. The pharmaceutical company website (listed below) for the manufacturer of telaprevir is helpful because it shows pictures of the various rash stages. Although it doesn't replace professional advice, it gives perspective.

Tips for managing dry skin and itching:

- Avoid scratching; if you must scratch, never use your fingernails or sharp objects. Try rubbing, vibration, or applying pressure instead of scratching. A good thing to "scratch" with is an ice cube.

- Drink plenty of water or other clear fluids to keep your entire body hydrated.
- Avoid extremely hot showers and baths.
- Apply moisturizer immediately after a shower or bath—before drying off with a towel. Creams are more effective moisturizers than lotions.
- Moisturize at least twice a day. There are many effective moisturizers; my two favorites are Trader Joe's Moisturizing Cream (extra dry formula) and A & D ointment for extremely dry skin. For dry hands, rub A & D on hands at bedtime and wear gloves to protect sheets from grease.
- Use nonperfumed, mild bath and personal care products.
- Avoid soap. Use a nonsoap cleanser such as Cetaphil or a similar substitute.
- Try oatmeal bath solution, baking soda, or unscented bath oils for bathing.
- Apply cold packs (wrapped in a thin towel) to the skin.
- Wear loose-fitting clothes made from natural fabrics that breathe.
- Protect your skin from the sun—wear sunscreen.
- Use lip balm with sunscreen to moisturize your lips.
- Keep rooms ventilated and at a temperature of 60°F to 70°F.
- For mild itching or rashes, ask your medical provider if you can use an over-the-counter topical hydrocortisone cream. Do not use hydrocortisone on your face or for prolonged periods unless directed to do so by your doctor.
- If rash or itching persist, talk to your medical provider about oral antihistamines such as over-the-counter diphenhydramine (Benadryl) or prescription-strength products such as hydroxyzine (Atarax) or topical steroids.

ADDITIONAL RESOURCES

www.incivek.com/hcp/assess-and-manage-rash

www.hcvadvocate.org/hepatitis/factsheets_pdf/SEM_Rashes.pdf

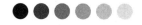

RESOURCES

BLOGS AND NEWS

HCV Advocate Blog, www.hcvadvocate.blogspot.com

HCV New Drug Research, www.hepatitiscnewdrugs.blogspot.com

Hepatitis C News, www.hepatitiscnews.com

Hep Blogs by Smart & Strong's HEP, www.blogs.hepmag.com

Lucinda K. Porter, www.LucindaPorterRN.com/blog

Medscape's Hepatitis C, www.medscape.com/resource/hepc

Your Best Friend's Guide to Hepatitis C, www.ihelpc.com

BRAIN FITNESS

For those with Internet access, type "puzzle," "games," or "brain games" into your search field and a world of opportunity will open up. There are game apps for smart phones and tablets, games on Facebook and other social media sites, and old-fashioned games such as cards and crossword puzzles. Here are a few to get you started:

www.gamesforthebrain.com

www.thinks.com/puzzles

CLINICAL TRIALS AND RESEARCH

CenterWatch, www.centerwatch.com

ClinicalTrials, www.clinicaltrials.gov

Clinical Trial Connection, www.clinicalconnection.com

HCV Advocate, www.hcvadvocate.org—Check out the *HCV Drug Pipeline* for updates on drugs in clinical trials. The factsheet, *Hepatitis C: Making Sense of Hepatitis C Research and Medical Literature* explains various aspects of research.

National Institutes of Health, www.nih.gov

COMPLEMENTARY AND ALTERNATIVE MEDICINE

ConsumerLab, www.consumerlab.com

Doc Misha's Chicken Soup Chinese Medicine, www.docmisha.com

Drug and Supplement Interaction Checker, www.drugs.com/drug_interactions.php

HCV Advocate, www.hcvadvocate.org—Look under the heading, Hepatitis C and Complementary and Alternative Medicine in the Fact Sheets section as well as the Herbal Glossary tab.

Memorial Sloan-Kettering Cancer Center, www.mskcc.org/aboutherbs

National Center for Complementary and Alternative Medicine's Hepatitis C and CAM, www.nccam.nih.gov/health/providers/digest

DISABILITY, DISCLOSURE, AND WORKPLACE ISSUES

Americans with Disabilities Act, www.ada.gov

HCV Advocate, www.hcvadvocate.org—Click on Benefits Column to learn more about insurance and disability benefits. The Factsheets section has information about disclosure and workplace issues.

Social Security, www.ssa.gov/disability

U.S. Department of Labor: Family and Medical Leave Act, www.dol.gov/whd/fmla/index.htm

FINANCIAL ISSUES AND MEDICAL INSURANCE

Medicare, www.medicare.gov

Needy Meds, www.needymeds.com

Partnership for Prescription Assistance, www.pparx.org

Patients Access Network Foundation, www.panfoundation.org

GENERAL HEALTH AND HEALTH IMPROVEMENT

Aetna Intelihealth, www.intelihealth.com

HealthFinder, www.healthfinder.gov

Mayo Clinic, www.mayoclinic.com

MedlinePlus, www.nlm.nih.gov/medlineplus

Merck Engage, www.merckengage.com

U.S. Department of Health and Human Services, www.hhs.gov

HEPATITIS C AND HIV/HCV CO-INFECTION INFORMATION

American Association for the Study of Liver Diseases, www.aasld.org/patients

American Liver Foundation, www.liverfoundation.org (800) GOLIVER/(800) 465-4837

Caring Ambassadors Hepatitis C Program, www.hepcchallenge.org

HCV Advocate, www.hcvadvocate.org

Health Pro, www.healthpro.us

HCVets, www.hcvets.com

Help4Hep, www.help4hep.org (877)HELP4HEP/(877) 435-7443

Hepatitis C Association, www.hepcassoc.org

Hep C Connection, www.hepc-connection.org

HepCBC, www.hepcbc.ca

Hep C Redefined, www.hepcredefined.com

Hepatitis Education Project, www.hepeducation.org

Hepatitis Foundation International, www.hepfi.org

HIV and Hepatitis, www.hivandhepatitis.com

National AIDS Treatment Advocacy Project, www.natap.org

National Alliance of State and Territorial AIDS Directors, www.nastad.org

National Viral Hepatitis Roundtable, www.nvhr.org

Project Inform, www.projectinform.org

Treatment Action Group, www.treatmentactiongroup.org

U.S. Department of Veterans Affairs Hepatitis C Information, www.hepatitis.va.gov

World Hepatitis Alliance, www.worldhepatitisalliance.org

HEPATITIS C TRANSMISSION/PREVENTION

Centers for Disease Control and Prevention, www.cdc.gov

Harm Reduction Coalition, www.harmreduction.org

HCV Advocate, www.hcvadvocate.org—Click on HCV Transmission and Prevention in the Factsheets section.

Hepatitis & Tattoos, www.hepatitistattoos.org

Sex and Hepatitis C, www.sexandhepc.com

HUMOR

Helpguide, www.helpguide.org/life/humor_laughter_health.htm

The Hepatitis Comics: Levity for the Liver, hepatitiscomics.blogspot.com

Laughter Heals Foundation, www.laughterheals.org

Laughter Therapy, www.laughtertherapy.com

Laughter Yoga, www.laughteryoga.org

YouTube, www.youtube.com

LAB TESTS

Labs On-Line, www.labtestsonline.org

MedlinePlus, www.nlm.nih.gov/medlineplus/laboratorytests.html

MEDITATION, STRESS REDUCTION, AND ANGER MANAGEMENT

The American Institute of Stress, www.stress.org

Anger Management Techniques, www.anger-management-techniques.org

Free Meditation Technique, www.freemeditations.com

Hep C Meditations, www.hepCmeditations.org—Free download of brief healthy liver recording and link to purchase meditation for a healthy liver CD

The Institute of Lifestyle Medicine, www.instituteoflifestylemedicine.org

Medline, www.nlm.nih.gov/medlineplus/stress.html

Stressbusting, www.stressbusting.co.uk

World Wide Online Meditation Center, www.meditationcenter.com

MENTAL HEALTH

HCV Advocate, www.hcvadvocate.org—Multiple articles about mental health and HCV, including "Coping with Depression and Hepatitis C"

Helpguide, www.helpguide.org

International Foundation for Research and Education for Depression, www.ifred.org—To find self-assessment tools and other information, click Understanding Depression.

Mayo Clinic, www.mayoclinic.com/health/ssris/MH00066—Link takes users to article about selective serotonin reuptake inhibitors (SSRIs). The rest of the website has more information on mental health.

Medline, www.nlm.nih.gov/medlineplus/depression.html—Click on links to other information.

Mental Health America, www.mentalhealthamerica.net

National Institute of Mental Health, www.nimh.nih.gov

NUTRITION

Harvard School of Public Health, www.hsph.harvard.edu/nutrition-source/index.html

Nutrition.gov, www.nutrition.gov

Oldways, www.oldwayspt.org

Slaying the Dragon with Food, www.squidoo.com/slaying-the-dragon—Foods that have 20 g or more of fat

PATIENT ADVOCACY

Hepatitis Prison Coalition, www.hcvinprison.org

Patient Advocate Foundation, www.patientadvocate.org

PHARMACEUTICAL COMPANIES

Companies with HCV Drugs in the Market

Genentech, manufacturer of peginterferon (Pegasys) and ribavirin (Copegus) www.pegasys.com (877) PEGASYS/(877) 734–2797

Kadmon Pharmaceuticals, manufacturer of ribavirin (Ribasphere) www.kadmon.com (888) 668–3393

Merck, manufacturer of peginterferon (PegIntron), ribavirin (Rebetol), and boceprevir (Victrelis), www.merck-cares.com

> www.pegintron.com
>
> www.victrelis.com
>
> (866) 939-HEPC/(866) 939–4372
>
> (800) 727–5400, Merck Patient Assistance Program—Provides free medicine for eligible patients.
>
> (866) 363–6379, Merck ACT program—Assists patients in finding coverage for medication.

Vertex, manufacturer of telaprevir (Incivek)
www.incivek.com (855)280–1650

Companies with HCV Drugs Applications under FDA Consideration

Gilead, www.gilead.com

Janssen, www.janssen.com

Companies with HCV Drugs in Mid-to-Late Phases of Development

AbbVie, www.abbvie.com

Achillion, www.achillion.com

Boehringer Ingelheim, www. boehringer-ingelheim.com

Bristol-Myers Squibb, www.bms.com

Idenix, www.idenix.com

PHYSICAL FITNESS

Centers for Disease Control's Exercise for Everyone, www.cdc.gov/physicalactivity/everyone/guidelines/index.html

President's Council on Fitness, Sports and Nutrition, www.fitness.gov

Shape Up America, www.shapeup.org

Squeeze It In, www.squeezeitin.com

YouTube, www.youtube.com

PREGNANCY AND CONTRACEPTION

Planned Parenthood, www.plannedparenthood.org

Ribavirin Pregnancy Registry—Registry for patients and their partners who become pregnant while taking ribavirin, http://ribavirinpregnancyregistry.com, (800) 593-2214

SIDE EFFECTS

Free from Hepatitis C: Your Complete Guide to Healing Hepatitis C by Lucinda K. Porter, RN, www.LucindaPorterRN.com

HCV Advocate, www.hcvadvocate.org—*A Guide to Hepatitis C: Treatment Side Effect Management* and other factsheets on this website.

Hep Drug Interactions, www.hep-druginteractions.org—Useful website for checking potential interactions between HCV medications and other drugs you may be taking.

SLEEP

American Academy of Sleep Medicine, www.yoursleep.aasmnet.org

American Sleep Association, www.sleepassociation.org

The National Sleep Foundation, www.sleepfoundation.org

STORYTELLING

HCV Advocate, www.hcvadvocate.org/community/stories.asp

StoryCorps, www.storycorps.org

World Hepatitis Alliance's Wall of Stories, www.worldhepatitisalliance.org/Community_Map/Real_Lives.aspx

SUBSTANCE AB USE AND RECOVERY

Alcoholic Anonymous (AA), (212) 870-3400,
www.alcoholics-anonymous.org

Centers for Disease Control and Prevention, www.cdc.gov/tobacco

Narcotic Anonymous (NA), (818) 773-9999, www.na.org

National Institute on Drug Abuse, www.nida.nih.gov

Substance Abuse and Mental Health Services Administration,
www.samhsa.gov

SUPPORT GROUPS—COMMUNITY AND WEB-BASED

Facebook—Enter "hepatitis C" in the search field.

Google Groups, www.groups.google.com—Enter "hepatitis C" in the
search field.

HCV Advocate, www.hcvadvocate.org—To find an HCV support
group meeting in your area, click on Support Groups. To start a support group, read the *Hepatitis C Support Group Manual* in the Factsheet
section

HCV Support, www.hcvsupport.org/forum/index.php

Hepatitis Central, www.hepatitis-central.com/hcv/support/main.html

National HCV Helpline, 877-HELP-4-HEP (877-435-7443)

Yahoo Groups, www.groups.yahoo.com—Enter "hepatitis C" in the
search field.

ACKNOWLEDGMENTS

A book is the accumulation of gifts received from many sources. To name them all would be like an ocean trying to thank every drop. However, there are a few acknowledgments that if I did not make them, I would lie awake at night with writer's remorse.

My first thank you is to my best friend, Deborah Appel. Although we learned grammar from the same public school teachers, evidently you paid attention. Deborah, thank you for teaching me about semicolons and making me look more competent than I really am.

I am deeply grateful to Stephany Evans, my agent at FinePrint Literary Management. I am truly fortunate to have you in my life. Thank you Demos Health for publishing this book. I am honored to work with Julia Pastore and the entire Demos Health team. You are magicians.

I owe a great debt to all the hepatitis C patients who made me a better nurse, and taught me how to manage the side effects of hepatitis C treatment. Thank you to my fellow heppers on Facebook, and a special thanks to Kim Young who gave permission to use her quote on Day 211.

My final appreciation is to my husband, Ed Porter. An author's spouse is the most neglected person in the world, yet you never complain. Although I have not yet dedicated a book to you, you deserve it. But I am saving that for another book. Thank you for your patience. especially if I neglect you again while writing the next book.

INDEX

abstain, 93
acceptance, 148
acetaminophen, 29, 93, 102
acupressure, 90, 105, 139
acupuncture, 90
ADA. *See* Americans with
    Disabilities Act
A & D ointment, 118, 141
affirmations, 97
agitation, 86
alanine aminotransferase (ALT), 93
alcohol, 93, 179
    avoiding, 141
    during HCV treatment, 27
ALT. *See* alanine aminotransferase
Ambien. *See* zolpidem
Americans with Disabilities Act
    (ADA), 13
anal/rectal discomfort, 35, 49
    managing, 207
anemia, 28, 45
anger, 86
    management, 67, 134, 147–148
antacid, 100
anti-anxiety medication, 35
antibiotics, 75
antidepressants, 35
antiviral, direct-acting, 36
antiviral medications, 57, 182, 184
anxiety, 41, 73, 79, 94, 104
    and fear, 191

apology, 93, 94
appetite, 37, 112
aromatherapy, 137
aspartate aminotransferase (AST), 93
aspirin, 29
AST. *See* aspartate aminotransferase
attitude, 167

Benadryl, 100, 210
biofeedback, 134
black tea, 89
blood-clotting ability, reduce, 77
blood transfusion, 28
boceprevir, 15, 18, 22, 36
body, preparing, 8–9
brain fog, 95, 113
breathing
    difficulties, 51
    exercises, 173
    problems, 118–119
    shortness of, 78

caffeine, 91
CAM. *See* complementary and
    alternative medicine
candidiasis, 75
CBC. *See* complete blood count
Cetaphil, 24
chamomile, 66

chaotic thoughts, 119
chemicals, hair color, 62
Chinese medicine, 70, 124, 134
cirrhosis, 15, 54, 55
communicable disease, 56
communication, 31
complementary and alternative
    medicine (CAM), 66
complete blood count (CBC), 47
confronting fear, 7–8
constipation, 19, 82
ConsumerLab.com, 71
coping skills, 115, 140
coping with pain, 69
courage, 192

DAAs. See Direct Antiviral Agents
dairy products, 86
dance therapy, 125, 171
daydreaming, 165, 187
dehydration, 19, 75, 124
depression, 60, 94, 104, 128
diabetes, 45
diarrhea, 19, 86
diet, 79, 136–137
dietary supplements, 57, 138
diphenhydramine. See Benadryl
Direct Antiviral Agents (DAAs), 12, 36
dizziness, 144
drugs, 40, 102
    avoiding, 141
    dosage of erectile dysfunction, 40
    erectile dysfunction, 16
    financial burden of, 45
    overuse of, 30
dry lips, 124
dry mouth remedies, 145
dryness, 22
dry skin, 161
    and itch, managing, 209–210

endurance, 105, 156, 191
erectile dysfunction drugs, 16
exercises, 68, 174
    qigong, 70, 180
    relaxation, 179
    stretching, 179
eye problems, 34

Facebook HCV groups, 191
fake cheerfulness, 157
fatigue, 22, 30, 32, 45, 58, 112, 129, 142,
    170, 183
    medical causes of, 70
fear
    anxiety and, 191
    confronting, 7–8
fever, 19
fibrosis, 55
financial preparations, HCV
    treatment, 14
fitness routine, 20–22
flu-like symptoms, 50
foggy thinking, 47
foods, fat, 205–206
forgiveness, 100
frustration, 47
ginger, 66

gratitude, 51–52, 108, 142, 190
    practice, 11, 161, 168

hair color chemicals, 62–63
hair loss, 61, 128, 157
hand washing, 56
happiness, improving immune
    system, 113
harmony, 81
HCV-positive organ, 182
HCV support group, 26
headaches, 30, 91, 166
healing, 91, 126, 160–161, 169
healing arts, 139
health, 152–153
    benefits of smiling, 130
    commitment to, 92
    maintenance, 91
health care, expectations of, 177, 178
health habits, 22
hemolytic anemia, 45
hemorrhoids, 76
herbs, 57, 82, 138–139
    herbal tea, 143
high-protein shakes, 37
hope, 185
human spirit and HCV treatment,
    121

humor, 10–11, 76, 101, 160, 165, 181–182
  health benefits of, 57
  laugh therapy, 69, 74, 90, 127, 177
hydration, 33, 102, 159, 170, 185
  intake of liquids, 89, 125, 149

ibuprofen, 29
imagination, 187
immune system, 28, 34, 48, 113
Imodium, 86
insomnia, 30, 39, 45, 60, 72, 84, 99, 115–116, 161
inspiration, 149
interferon. *See* peginterferon
Internet, 38
irritability, 41
isolation, 101
itching, 50, 55, 72, 99, 130, 209–210

lab tests, 44
language and thought, 133
lavender oil
  for headaches, 137
  and insomnia, 116
lightheadedness, 42–43
lips, dry, 124
liquids, intake of, 89, 125, 149
loneliness, 107, 119–120, 135–136, 151–152
loss of appetite, 112

"magic mouthwash," 100
massage, 101
medical appointments, 32, 44
medical care, 19
medical problems, 150
medications, 19, 34, 36, 75
  anti-anxiety, 35
  antiviral, 57, 182, 184
  to control itching, 55
  HCV, 19, 20, 34, 66
  oral, 25
  psychiatric, 58
  side effects of, 165–166

meditation, 11, 78, 133, 134
memory loss, 136
Metamucil. *See* psyllium
migraines, 30, 91
milk thistle, 71, 82
mind–body spiritual practice, 69
mindfulness, 186
mind, preparing, 9–10
MiraLax. *See* polyethylene glycol 3350
moodiness, 79
mood-management medication, 94
motivation, 149
mouth sores, 53–54
mucous membranes, 53
music and HCV treatment, 96

napping, 70
naproxen, 29
nature and HCV treatment, 59, 118
nausea, 41, 66
negative attitude, 140
negative self-talk, 115, 156
neuropsychiatric side effects, 58
nutrition. *See* diet

online hepatitis C groups, 87, 120
oral hygiene, 74
oral infections, 74
organ donation, 182

pain, 100, 102, 123, 161
  coping with, 69
  distraction for, 131
  humor, 137
  management and HCV treatment, 122–123
patience, 52–53, 158, 176, 178, 183, 188
peginterferon, 22, 48, 133, 200, 201
  injection, 106
  self-injection of, 17
petroleum jelly, 141
photosensitivity, 32
physical fitness, 48
pleasure, during HCV treatment, 123, 145–146, 150–151, 186
polyethylene glycol 3350, 76

positive thinking, 140, 146
post-treatment recovery period, key
    issues for, 196
protocol for HCV treatment, 14–15
psychiatric medications, 58
psychiatric side effects, 16
psychological resilience, 117
psyllium, 76

qigong exercise, 70, 116, 157, 170, 180

rashes, 72, 209–210
raspberry leaf tea, 66
rebound headache, 30
red blood cells, 46, 47
relaxation exercises, 96, 179
respiratory problems, 78
responder-relapsers, 198
response–guided therapy, 63
results, treatment, 195–198
ribavirin, 18, 22, 28, 45, 57, 200, 201

safety, 86
saliva production, 108
self-absorption, 96
self-administering injections, 25
self-injection
    appointment to review, 25
    of peginterferon, 17
    psychological component to
        overcome, 21
self-pity, 151
sex, health, 162
sexual dysfunction, 83
sexual problems, 40, 114, 137–138
shortness of breath, 78
short-temperedness, 41
side effects, 93, 106, 117–118,
        130, 153
    of HCV medications, 166
    of HCV treatment, 23–24, 28, 30–32,
        72, 77, 84, 156
        fatigue, 156
        hydration, 170

insomnia, 30, 39
management, 138, 140–141
nausea, 41
preparing for, 15–16
simeprevir, 200
skin problems, managing, 209–210
sleep
    interrupters, 163
    problems, 72
    quality and amount of, 163
sleep hygiene, 24, 53
smiling, health benefits of, 130
sofosbuvir, 200
spiritual health, 114
spiritual practice, 11
St. John's wort, 16
stomach pain, 19
stool softener, 76
stress, 75, 144, 167–168
    management, 67
    reduction techniques, 77
    relieving techniques, 124
stretching exercises, 179
support groups, 13–14, 26
support system, 42
    setting up, 13–14

telaprevir, 15, 16, 18, 22, 35, 36, 205, 209
thought, language and, 133
thrush, 74, 75
thyroid, 45
    abnormalities, evaluating, 184
tiredness. *See* fatigue
treatment, HCV
    all-encompassing nature of, 165
    completion of, 155
    getting organized for,
        11–12
    learning about, 5–7
    managing, 12
    preparing others, 12–13
treatment-related mood changes, 34
Tylenol. *See* acetaminophen
valerian, 72
viral load, HCV, 198
vision problems, 34, 121

visualization, 139
  power of, 38
  on side effects, 39
vitamin D, 40
vomiting, 19

walking, 20, 122
water, intake of, 102, 125, 149, 170

web-based support groups, 38
websites for information and
    support, 120, 132
weight gain, 132
weight loss, 112

zolpidem, 16

ABOUT THE AUTHOR

Lucinda K. Porter, RN, is an advocate, nurse, health educator, and patient devoted to increasing awareness about hepatitis C. She is the author of *Free from Hepatitis C* and writes for the *HCV Advocate* among other publications. Porter was named the Top Social HealthMaker in hepatitis C by Sharecare. She lives in Grass Valley, California.

www.LucindaPorterRN.com